TRANSFORM Your Health
TRANSFORM Your Life

How you can TRANSFORM your life mentally, physically, spiritually, socially, and financially

By David W. Sloan,
MH, PhD, DNM, RNT

TEACH Services, Inc.
PUBLISHING
www.TEACHServices.com • (800) 367-1844

World rights reserved. This book or any portion thereof may not be copied or reproduced in any form or manner whatever, except as provided by law, without the written permission of the publisher, except by a reviewer who may quote brief passages in a review.

The author assumes full responsibility for the accuracy of all facts and quotations as cited in this book. The opinions expressed in this book are the author's personal views and interpretations, and do not necessarily reflect those of the publisher.

This book is provided with the understanding that the publisher is not engaged in giving spiritual, legal, medical, or other professional advice. If authoritative advice is needed, the reader should seek the counsel of a competent professional.

Copyright © 2022 David W. Sloan
Copyright © 2022 TEACH Services, Inc.
ISBN-13: 978-1-4796-1401-1 (Paperback)
ISBN-13: 978-1-4796-1402-8 (ePub)
Library of Congress Control Number: 2022903318

All emphasis in Scripture quotations is supplied by the author.

All Scripture quotations, unless otherwise indicated, are taken from the New King James Version®. Copyright © 1990 by Thomas Nelson. Used by permission. All rights reserved.

Scripture quotations marked NIV are taken from the New International Version. Copyright © 1973, 1978, 1984, 2011 by Biblica, Inc®. Used by permission. All rights reserved worldwide.

Scripture quotations marked NLT are taken from the New Living Translation. Copyright © 1996, 2004, 2015 by Tyndale House Foundation. Used by permission of Tyndale House Publishers, Inc., Carol Stream, Illinois 60188. All rights reserved.

Scripture quotations marked KJV are taken from the King James Version®. Public domain.

Scripture quotations marked ESV are taken from the English Standard Version. Copyright © 2001 by Crossway, a publishing ministry of Good News Publishers. Used by permission. All rights reserved.

Scripture quotations marked BSB are taken from The Holy Bible, Berean Study Bible. Copyright © 2016, 2018 by Bible Hub. Used by permission. All rights reserved worldwide.

Scripture quotations marked AMP are taken from the Amplified Bible. Copyright © 2015 by the Lockman Foundation. Used by permission.

MEDICAL/LEGAL/FINANCIAL DISCLAIMER. Any counsel made by Dr. Sloan in this book is not to be used to diagnose or treat any illness, condition, or disease. His advice, suggestions, protocols, and supplement recommendations should be considered only after seeking the advice of a registered healthcare practitioner. Dr. Sloan will in no instance be held responsible or liable for any untoward results, side effects, illness, or disease resulting from the use of any of his dietary, lifestyle, or supplementary protocols. For the diagnosis of any ailment or disease, psychological or psychiatric disorder, please consult a licensed physician.

Dr. Sloan is not a financial planner or advisor and will not be held liable or responsible in any way for any financial strategies, purchases, investments, etc. that the reader may decide to make. Dr. Sloan's recommendations are strictly for general informational and educational purposes. For your own financial planning or advice, please consult a qualified financial advisor.

All attempts have been made to verify information that is provided in this book and its ancillary materials. Neither the author nor publisher assumes any responsibility for errors, inaccuracies, or omissions and is not responsible for any loss by the reader in any manner. Any slights of people or organizations are unintentional. All efforts to correct any issues will be made in the next printing of the book.

TEACH Services, Inc.
P U B L I S H I N G
www.TEACHServices.com • (800) 367-1844

Table of Contents

Foreword 7
Acknowledgements. 8
Note to Reader 9
Only Two Years to Live!. 11
T-R-A-N-S-F-O-R-M 17
T is for … Trust in the Lord. 21
R is for … Rest 35
A is for … Activity 48
N is for … Nutrition 64
S is for … Supplementation. 77
F is for … Finances. 95
O is for … Outlook. 104
R is for … Relationships 117
M is for … Motivation 125
Conclusion. 141
Bibliography 144

Foreword

by Bill Santos, executive director and founder of Lessons for Living Ministries

"I have known Dr. Sloan for the better part of 15 years and I have come to know him as someone who is genuinely concerned with the well-being of others. I know he never thought he would play such a vital role in helping others improve their health, but a sobering medical diagnosis at a young age became the impetus for him to better understand his body and how to get the most out of it. That learning has helped thousands improve their lives and maximize the health potential of their bodies. I have interviewed Dr. Sloan many times on my television program and his interviews have consistently been some of the highest viewed programs, live and later on social media. Why? Because he cares and the information he provides is understandable and practical. I have no doubt that you will benefit greatly from the knowledge that Dr. Sloan has acquired over the years. The TRANSFORM acronym is genius to help us remember and implement the practical lessons that lead to better health. I encourage you to learn the lessons and more importantly adopt them into your life, so you too can TRANSFORM your Health and Your Life!"

Acknowledgements

First and foremost, I acknowledge the oversight of this book by my Savior, Jesus Christ, who I surrendered my heart to many decades ago. He has been there constantly to patiently guide me along this life's journey. He has blessed me with remarkable success in treating tens of thousands of patients solely using natural medicines and treatments. By God's grace, I have been able to deliver my patients from pain, suffering, and poor health into optimal, extraordinary, and often life-changing wellness and vitality. It is through Him, and the outpouring of His Holy Spirit that has been of inestimable value and support to me, that I have been able to bring this important information together for my Christian and non-Christian readers alike. Jesus, my gratitude for what You have done for me knows no bounds—You are my all in all.

To my wife Erika, who for well over forty years has stood by me with unwavering love and support. Words cannot describe how much this has meant to me. Thank you for being my wife, the mother of our three sons, and my best friend.

Thanks to Michelle Post who provided the opportunity, encouragement, and know-how for me to finally get this book written.

Note to Reader

Although this book is focused on targeting the Christian community, my intention is by no means to exclude anyone. I would very much like to encourage those who are of other spiritual beliefs or faith as well as those who espouse no particular spiritual leanings to also read this book. I am confident that in it you will find many things of great value in equipping yourself to enjoy optimal health. My hope and prayer is that it will be a great blessing to everyone.

— Dr. David Sloan

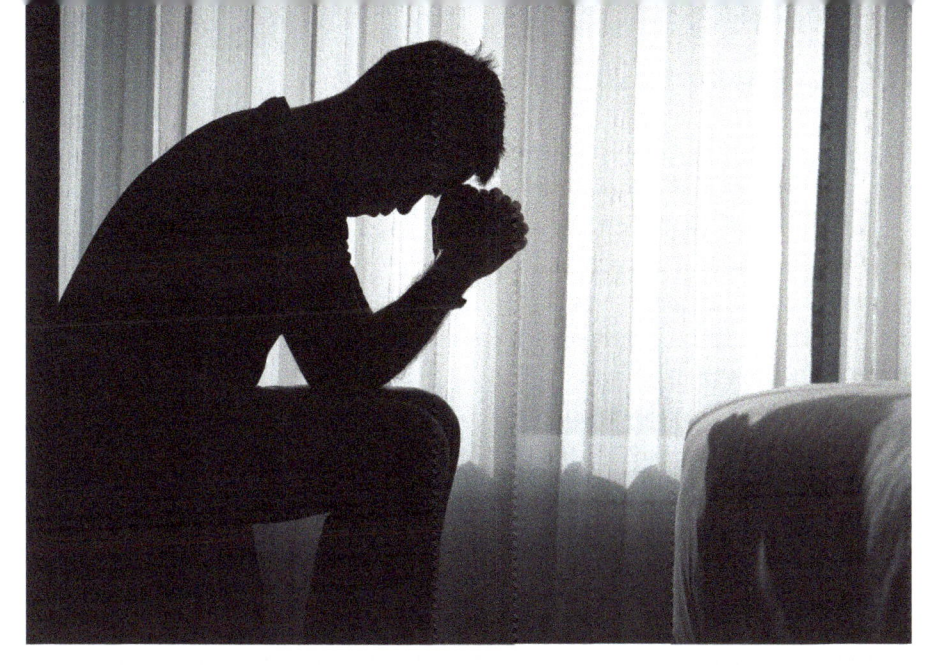

Only Two Years to Live!

"You probably don't have more than two years to live!"

What a shock to hear this from a holistic doctor whom I respected and trusted. I had just been married a year and couldn't picture myself sharing this horrible news with my beautiful bride. With my whole life in front of me, how could it be that at just twenty-four years of age, I would soon be exiting this planet?

I knew I wasn't well and hadn't been since childhood. I was now in my twenties, a rock musician continually touring across Canada, and even though I never once missed a performance, I pretty much knew every walk-in clinic in every town and city we performed in.

> *"You probably don't have more than two years to live!" What a shock to hear this from a holistic doctor whom I respected and trusted.*

I was experiencing more difficulties than just a sore throat or infected sinus or bronchioles. I had trouble digesting my food. I had gas and bloating. I was constipated. At times I could not breathe and had chest pains around my heart. I also had bladder and prostate issues, lower back pain, sleep deprivation, low energy, and low immunity. I was in terrible shape. One night, in Calgary, Alberta, as we were playing on stage, our bass player Gerry collapsed from severe exhaustion right before our very eyes.

As we helped him down to a table to recover, I wondered if I would be next. Was I destined to be another burnt-out rock musician?

I went to my family doctor for a physical. I complained that I was sick nearly all the time. He ran a series of blood tests and much to my disbelief, pronounced me in good health. If this was good health, I wondered what bad health might be. I left his office extremely perplexed and with many more questions than answers.

Some real answers were to come soon. A friend introduced me to Dr. Randy Hardy, who was not only a chiropractor but a naturopath as well. Hmmm, I thought to myself, could this doctor possibly be someone who could help me?

During my appointment with him, Dr. Hardy explained to me that much of my body was inflamed and slowly but surely all the major systems were deteriorating and beginning to shut down, hence the two-year timeline. This included my respiratory system, digestive system, cardiovascular system, musculoskeletal system, and immune system. Despite the bleak diagnosis, he told me that if I were to make significant changes to my diet and lifestyle, he was optimistic that I could turn this situation around. "You will need to change to a vegan diet. This is the foundation of your treatment. I will give you two herbs, myrrh and slippery elm bark, which you are to take every day in the form of teas."

The next day I went instantly from being a high-fat, sugar, junk food, milk, meat and potatoes type of guy to a complete vegan (plant-based) diet, shunning all meat, poultry, fish, eggs, all dairy products, sugar, candy and other sweets, desserts, table salt, fried foods, foods in "crinkly packages," soft drinks, caffeinated beverages, fast food, white flour, commercial salad dressings, and any other processed items.

"What food is there left that you can eat?" I remember my wife asking me. It was true; my choices were rather limited. But it wasn't as if I had much choice. If I wanted to beat that prognosis, I needed to make radical changes. I thankfully sat down to the first of many, many meals consisting of a baked potato, some steamed vegetables, and lots of raw greens.

I followed Dr. Randy's instructions religiously. We were basically lost for a while as to the vegan (plant-based) way of life—and forget it if I wanted to dine out and splurge. My staple fare at a restaurant for some time was the same—a baked potato, steamed or sautéed vegetables, and salad. Mercifully, more and more plant-based choices became available at restaurants as the months and years passed.

In just a few weeks or so, I began to feel a difference. I could tell that I was on the right track. For one thing, my constant plugged nasal passages cleared up. One day as a few of my band mates and I were shopping, I could actually smell bananas. My sense of smell had been pretty much defunct for years and now it was just amazing to be able to smell again, especially since the bananas were not just in the aisle before me but a full two aisles over. My family will tell you that I still have the sharpest sense of smell of anyone they know today—many years later.

Most of my allergy and respiratory problems were behind me and I rarely got sick again. This was a revolutionary experience, let me tell you. I started to feel well enough to start jogging and doing sit-ups and push-ups while touring with the band. I brought along a little cookstove and made all my own meals. Jim, the drummer who I roomed with, got to see what a health fanatic I had become. I began to feel so much better that I started to become very interested in natural and nutritional ways of wellness. I visited every book section of every health food store along the way, developing a very formidable holistic health library. Poring over every word, I came to know these books backwards and forwards.

It became evident, however, that my complete recovery wasn't going to be quite that quick and easy. In fact, there were certain issues that were deeply entrenched and chronic. I had by then figured out that dairy foods were actually the fundamental cause of all the congestion and mucus buildup in my respiratory system. To learn that the foods that I grew up loving were causing a lot of my health issues was a troubling and rather devastating discovery for me. I began to wonder what other foods and substances might be mischief makers for me.

A year or so had passed and by then, through a remarkable encounter with Jesus Christ, I was gradually led out of rock music and at the same time was blessed by an amazing transformation through nutrition.

My whole perspective on life was changed forever. In many ways, what I was brought up to believe about numerous things was challenged. I often came to the conclusion that what the majority thought was right, acceptable, or okay, wasn't actually right at all.

So, what do I mean by that? Well, for starters, the Lord was now making it clear to me that as a rock musician, I was not serving God by getting up there singing about a "gin-soaked bar room queen in Memphis"[1] and other such things! Neither was I serving Him when I realized that through my music, I was encouraging people to get drunk, get stoned, and engage in all kinds of reckless behavior leading to acts of violence (we witnessed

---

1   The Rolling Stones, Jagger-Richards, "Honky Tonk Women," June 1969; London Records (US), released July 4, 1969, as a non-album single.

many a knock 'em down, drag 'em out fight), unwanted pregnancies, infidelity, and potential deaths due to drunk driving.

Other things that I had never thought of before began to concern me. Take, for example, the fact that my ears would be ringing for weeks after we took a rare break from touring or how thick the smoke was in the room that I was breathing in for hours on end every night. These were the days before air filters and before smoking was banned in clubs.

It came to the point that I could clearly see I was in the devil's playground and Satan was using me to achieve his ends. How terrible I felt as that realization gradually dawned on me.

There was more. As mentioned earlier, after being a meat-lover for the first twenty-odd years of my life, I was now a ... vegan. What a strange turn of events. During this time, I had read a lot about why a plant-based diet was superior on many different levels—physically, mentally, and spiritually, yet this was certainly not popular at the time like it is now. Most people we talked to about our dietary change were horrified and worried about us and how we could live without meat. As it was, the husband of one of these well-meaning persons was a heavy meat-eater. Sadly, his diet and lifestyle were most likely responsible for an early death in his mid-fifties. Had I been able to successfully advise him and so many others around us, undoubtedly, they would have lived many more years.

As I mentioned above, the cleaning up of my diet led me to improve in so many ways, the most significant of which was spiritually. Being brought up a pastor's kid was now coming back to me and I credit my parents with investing in the time and energy to see to it that I knew about Jesus, who He was, and the ultimate sacrifice He made for me.

Now it meant something to me, and I was drawn to find out more about who this Jesus really was. This led my wife and I on a spiritual journey that took us from our mainline Protestant church to studying with Pentecostals, Baptists, Jehovah's Witnesses, and Seventh-day Adventists. The Lord had given me sufficient experience in seeing and reading firsthand about the occult, New Age, and esoteric philosophies and many derivatives of these. The Lord made it clear that I was not to get involved with that.

In time, through the remarkable leading of the Lord, we were unmistakably directed to the Seventh-day Adventist Church. This was the body of Christ's believers that we were to become a part of. It truly is a church with a special message for these last days before Christ's second coming. Much of my present worldview has been shaped by the clear biblical teachings that this church has opened my eyes to understand so well.

God was impressing me to look at a career in natural medicine and nutritional counseling. If this could help me so dramatically, I thought, just imagine how I could help many, many others with their health issues. This potential consumed me and thus began an unquenchable thirst for training in the nutritional and herbal field. On Dr. Randy's advice, I eventually achieved my master herbalist degree. I began a course in clinical nutrition, in which I ended up completing my PhD. I started a humble practice in 1980 in the living room of our small apartment.

Most of my respiratory, cardiovascular, and immune issues were clearing up, but I still struggled with my digestion and elimination. I suffered from gas, bloating, abdominal pain, and irregular elimination, plus a nagging pain in the right testicle. I had heard about an herbalist by the name of John Finch in London, Ontario, who was doing great things with his patients, so I booked an appointment with him. After an intensive assessment, he introduced me to the concept of body cleansing and detoxifying. Thus, began a journey that was to involve many different types of herbal and homeopathic formulas, probiotics, candida treatment, vermifuges (antiparasitic herbs), fasting, colonics, and medical foods that he conceived of himself—quite remarkable and very much ahead of his time. Over time, as my digestion and elimination improved, I began to feel much better. I took more courses and training and later that year was certified in colon hydrotherapy by Dr. Robert A. Wood, the father of colon therapy.

So here I am, over forty years later and still very much alive. I am so thankful to God for leading me to these and numerous other wonderful natural health practitioners and for the restorative power of nutrition. We have raised three strong and healthy sons the natural, nutritional way and they in turn are doing the same with our grandchildren. I have the energy to keep up with and often exceed those half my age. I have been privileged to have successfully helped tens of thousands of patients over the years and that is reward enough. However, it took three to four years of continuous hard work at rebuilding my health and I still must work at it to this day. Much of my own experience being sick with so many disorders has helped me to develop empathy, confidence, and skill at knowing how to deal with others' illnesses. Out of my health challenges came a career—a life's work of fulfillment and joy at helping others get well ... really well again!

I am excited that you have decided to go on this journey with me to TRANSFORM *your* health. God has been gracious to have shown me many health secrets, some of which I have included in the pages of this book. The Lord has truly blessed me with optimal health over all these years and in turn I want to share some of these fundamentals that you can implement into your life ... today!

I truly believe that if you endeavor to follow the principles given in this acronym—TRANSFORM—it will not only TRANSFORM your health, but it will also TRANSFORM your life.

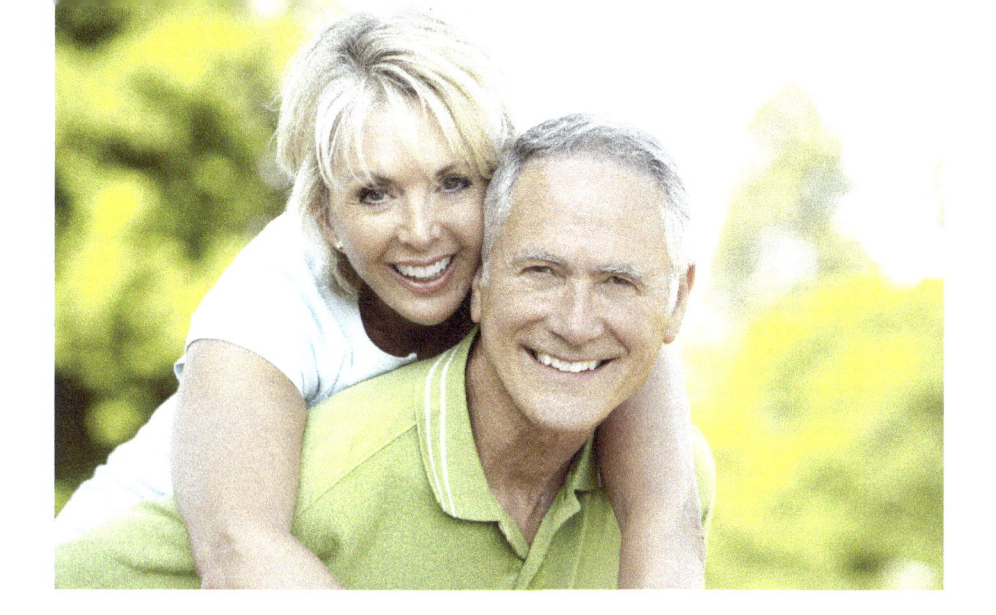

T-R-A-N-S-F-O-R-M

So, how did I come up with this word, TRANSFORM, to represent what is needed to be optimally healthy in the twenty-first century? As a registered natural health practitioner since 1980 when I began my full-time practice, I have been asked on many occasions to speak to different groups on health.

One day just a few years ago, I was thinking about how I could impart the health and life principles that I have learned to live by—principles that have made such a difference in not only my own health but in the health of my family, friends, and tens of thousands of patients over the years. I started to write down a few things. What if I could come up with an acronym that would truly reflect what I believe makes up optimal health in this modern, technological, and informational age we live in?

In an amazing and clear revelation that only God can give, the word TRANSFORM appeared in my mind and I wrote it down. Then I looked at what each letter might stand for: T—Trust in the Lord. That's a good place to start. Now what about R? Hmmm … Rest. Alright. A—Activity. And in minutes I had my health acronym that I know was a gift from God.

Let's look at the health/life principles that this acronym stands for:

T—Trust in the Lord

R—Rest

A—Activity

N—Nutrition

S—Supplementation

F—Finances

O—Outlook

R—Relationships

M—Motivation

 Each of the next nine chapters will be dedicated to these principles one at a time. But before you jump into the first letter—Trust in the Lord, I highly recommend that you do the Balance Wheel of Life exercise first. Here is what I want you to do.
 On a blank sheet of paper put a dot in the center. Now draw a 3-inch horizontal straight line from this dot to the right. This line will represent a "spoke" in your wheel of life that would be a score of 10. You will use this line as a guide on how long to draw your other "spokes." Take each letter from the word TRANSFORM and rate yourself on how strong you are in this area on a scale of 1 to 10—10 being the highest and best score. For example, if you are rating yourself on Trust in the Lord and you give yourself a score of 5, then draw a line out from the center approximately

about half the length of the 3-inch guideline (which represents a perfect score of 10) that you drew earlier. On that line write "Trust."

See Fig. 1 which is an illustration of a "perfect" Balance Wheel of Life and Fig. 2 which illustrates how a person's might look when completed.

Here is the diagram of a perfect Balance Wheel of Life.

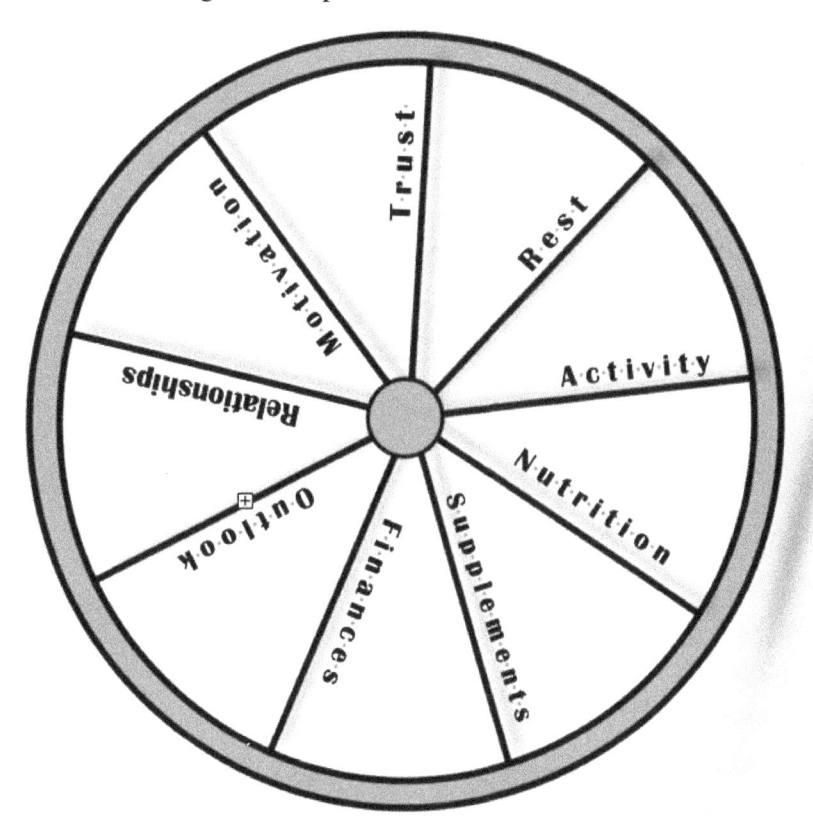

Fig. 1

Each letter from the word TRANSFORM will be a spoke coming out from the dot you have placed in the center so that when you are done rating yourself, you will have 9 spokes coming out from the center much like the spokes of a bicycle wheel. My suggestion is that if you are not certain on how to rate yourself on a certain letter, you can jump ahead in the book to that chapter, read it, and then come back to finish that "spoke."

To complete the wheel, draw a line connecting each "spoke" until you have what resembles a wheel. Don't be discouraged if your wheel looks rather misshapen—we all need to start somewhere. This exercise will clearly show you where your strengths and weaknesses lie in your Balance Wheel of Life. Date it at the top and keep it somewhere where you can refer to it three months, six months, a year from now and then redo a new one every so often and compare your results. A great time would be to do it every January 1st as you look ahead to what you feel the Lord is impressing you to work on or achieve in all these areas for the coming year.

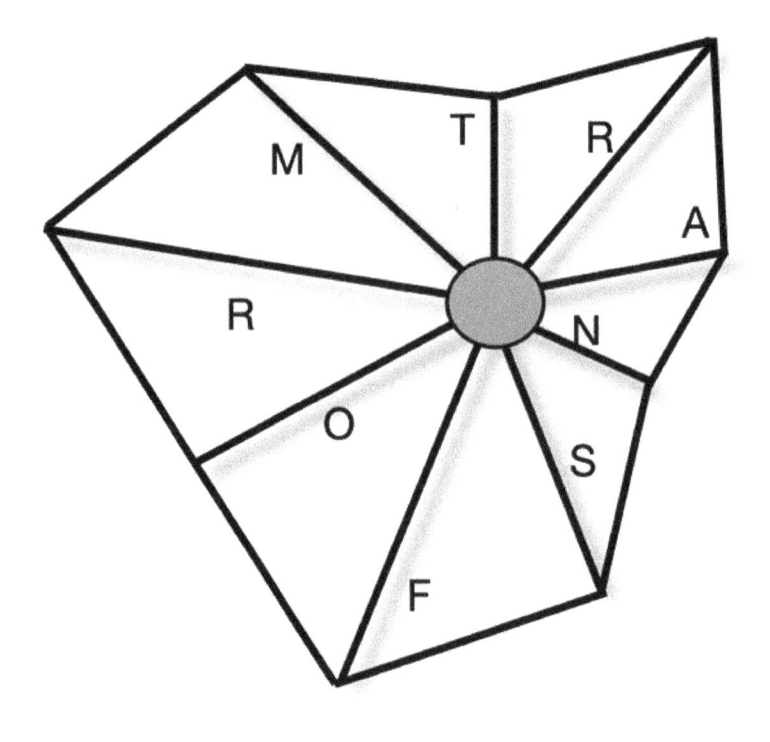

Fig. 2

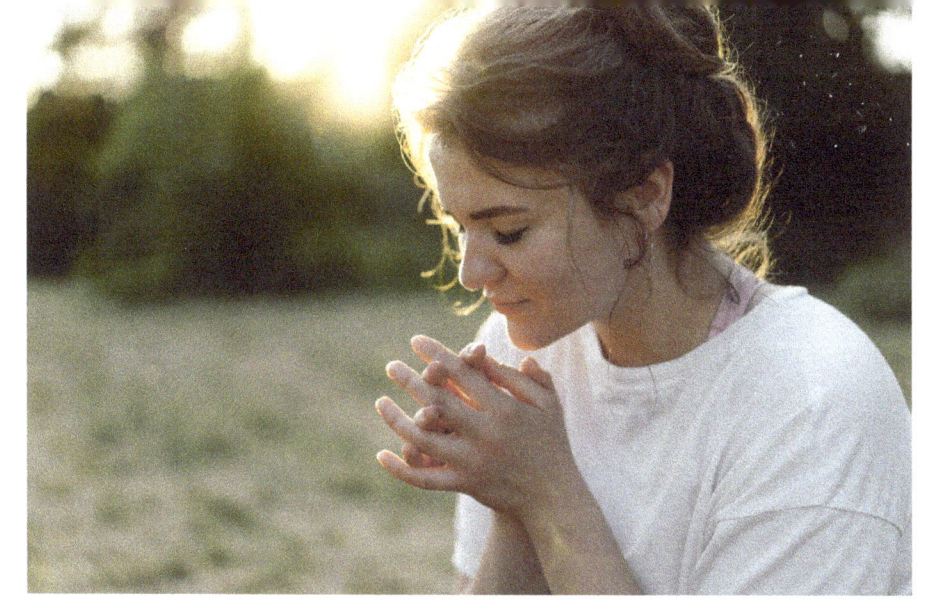

T is for … Trust in the Lord

"Trust in the LORD with all your heart, and lean not on your own understanding; in all your ways acknowledge Him, and He shall direct your paths" (Prov. 3:5–6).

The first letter in the acronym TRANSFORM stands for **Trust in the Lord.** In all that we do, we need to consider this as coming first in any of our attempts to transform our lives. Trust in God is the key that unlocks the door to a more powerful, confident, amazing, and vibrant life!

The well-known Scripture passage from Proverbs carries a depth of action that is much more than meets the eye, however. It means surrendering not part of, but all of our heart, mind, and body to Him—all of our hopes, dreams, desires, aspirations, goals … everything! Another word for trust is faith. When we know that God is in control of our lives and everything that goes on in our world and beyond, we can rest assured that He is for us. "What shall we then say to these things? If God be for us, who can be against us?" (Rom. 8:31, KJV). Jesus said, "I am the bread of life. He who comes to Me shall never hunger …. [A]nd the one who comes to Me I will by no means cast out" (John 6:35, 37).

You may wonder where or how we come up with this faith or trust that I am talking about. Not to worry. The Lord has already provided us with the gift of faith. It says in the Bible in Romans 12:3, "God has dealt to *each one a measure of faith*" (emphasis supplied). It is this "seed" of faith with which He has gifted us that we are to grow in faith and trust.

In Romans 10:17, we read, "[s]o then faith *comes* by hearing, and hearing by the word of God."

What is this "word of God" exactly? Well, most people when asked this question would say that it is the Bible. And they would be partially correct, but it goes much deeper than that. If we turn to the first chapter of John in the Bible and read the first verse, it says, "In the beginning was the Word, and the Word was with God, and the Word was God" (John 1:1, NIV, emphasis supplied). We discover from this that Jesus, God's Son, is described as the "Word." So, being the "Word," Jesus provided us with the Bible which I like to say is the complete instruction manual or guidebook on how we are to live. In 2 Timothy 3:16–17, NLT, the Bible says: "All Scripture is inspired by God and is useful to teach us what is true and to make us realize what is wrong in our lives. It corrects us when we are wrong and teaches us to do what is right. God uses it to prepare and equip his people to do every good work."

Jesus was with God in the beginning and is described as an equal to God. Isn't that interesting? This clearly puts to rest the argument claiming that although Jesus was a great teacher and spiritual leader, He was just a created being, a highly spiritually developed man. No, the Bible clearly calls him God, which along with the Holy Spirit makes up the Godhead—the three in one God.

Let's look a little further at John chapter 1 and verses 2 and 3, NIV. "He was with God in the beginning. Through Him all things were made; without Him nothing was made that has been made." So, here we see that not only was Jesus an equal part of the Godhead, but He was our Creator—the Creator of the universe, in fact!

So, when we trust in the Lord, we can fully put our trust in Jesus because He is the one who created us and He knows us intimately inside and out. He knows everything about us, what we like, what we don't like, our fears, our joys, our worries, challenges, frustrations ... everything!

Not only that, but He cares for us with a love that knows no bounds. Jeremiah 31:3, NLT, says, "Long ago the LORD said to Israel [Christians are modern-day Israel—God's people]: 'I have loved you, my people, with an everlasting love. With unfailing love I have drawn you to myself.'"

In my own experience over the forty-plus years as a natural health practitioner, I have had to really learn what it means to trust in God's provision for me and my family. My wife and I pledged that she would stay home and raise our three sons. This, of course, meant that our total income would come entirely from my practice. I worked very hard to build up our clientele but at the end of the day it was the Lord who I needed to depend on to bring patients to me.

For example, many, many times, I would check my schedule for the next day and I would see that it was not busy at all, with hardly any patients booked in. As has been my habit, I would include in my prayers a request for more new patients, that we would be busier, see more patients and receive more sales of products that day than I would ever expect possible. Miraculously, at the end of that day, the amount of business always was far more than we ever expected. It was always a clear sign from God that He would stoop to answer my prayers and that has always been so humbling. In all these years, His provision for us has never failed, and on top of that, He has granted me amazing success at getting people well again. What a blessing this has been to witness His grace to me, my wife, and our family firsthand.

Look for the small miracles in your day. Even write them down. You will be surprised how many things work out even though you *didn't even ask*. You will come to know your Creator on a more intimate level—a Savior who cares about us and loves us so much that even the little, seemingly insignificant things are important to Him! You can look forward to what He is about to do in your life today and every day.

> *Look for the small miracles in your day. Even write them down. You will be surprised how many things work out even though you didn't even ask.*

Having related the uncanny way in which the Lord ostensibly answered my prayers within hours or less, I wouldn't want you to think that God is like some supernatural bellhop who is just waiting to be at your beck and call for every whim that crosses your mind.

My requests have always been prefaced by saying, "If it is according to Your will, O Lord." Our trust in God is rooted in a sense that He knows what is best for us and we accept what happens, regardless of whether our prayers were answered or not—or answered differently from the way we thought they should be.

I believe God always answers prayer but, in His time, *not ours*. I remember our eldest son wanted to attend a Christian school. He had just completed ninth grade at our local high school, and we had wanted to wait to send him to a Christian high school until grades eleven, twelve, and thirteen (still had grade thirteen at the time).

With *him* requesting to go, rather than the other way around, we felt we needed to support his desire. The only drawback was that the school was more than two hours away by car and he would have to live on campus in the boys' dorm. We weren't comfortable with our son living so far away in these important teen years, so we sent him off but put our house up for sale in the meantime.

As soon as the house sold, we would look for a home close to the school. We fully expected the Lord would sell our house very quickly because, after all, surely it was God's will that our son attend a Christian school and be able to live at home with his parents. Well, the months went by and nothing. We changed realtors, we tried different things, but no sale. After his first semester, he told us he wanted to come home. He was doing well, getting high grades, and loved everything about the school except he was having major challenges living at the dorm. What a time! A real answer to prayer came when one of his teachers offered to put him up at their home. This was a turning point for Derek and from then on, he flourished at the school and was a top student all the way through. Meanwhile, our house was still not selling.

Finally, we received a good offer and were able to move. It took *more than a whole year* to sell, but looking back, I see how many miracles had to take place in order for us to make this exodus.

I had a very busy practice and was working in three clinics at the time. It was a very complex situation, but the Lord pulled all the strings. The timing was intricately and masterfully orchestrated. The amazing way in which the Lord led us to the home we purchased would not have happened if our other home sold earlier because our new home was not put on the market until *the very day* we came to the city to find a new home.

We were unmistakably led to this house that, incredibly, satisfied our long wish list and we *still* live in the same house today, almost twenty years later. God is so good!

A very dear Scripture of mine that illustrates perfectly what is going on with my experience described above is Jeremiah 29:11–14, NIV. This passage will strengthen your trust in God that He has your best interest in mind. "'For I know the plans I have for you,' declares the LORD, 'plans to prosper you and not to harm you, plans to give you hope and a future. Then you will call on me and come and pray to me, and I will listen to you. You will seek me and find me when you seek me with all your heart. I will be found by you,' declares the LORD."

Of course, the greatest test to our trusting in the Lord happens when our faith comes under fire—when disaster, tragedy, or tough times befall us. When a little child is murdered or a mother dies of breast cancer or an elderly woman is robbed and badly beaten, or a terrorist shooter opens fire in a classroom killing many innocent children, we are often left asking the question "Why?" Why would a loving God allow this to happen or worse, cause this to occur?

As we develop our faith in God over time, through prayer, meditation, and Bible study, we will mature in our understanding of what is actually going on.

Sin entered the world when Adam and Eve disobeyed God. In Genesis, the first book of the Bible, we are introduced to Lucifer who was the beautiful, perfect, and wise covering cherub. This was a very high position in God's hierarchy, where Lucifer's wings shielded God's throne (Ezek. 28:16). In time, he allowed pride to enter his heart and considered himself equal to God.

Lucifer convinced one-third of the heavenly angels to side with him and unbelievably, they decided to rebel against God. There was war in heaven and Michael, the archangel (Jesus Himself), and His angels prevailed. Lucifer, who was now renamed Satan, "that old serpent, who is the devil, Satan" (Rev. 20:2, NLT), was defeated and cast down from heaven to earth for a time. You can read all of this in the seventeenth chapter of Revelation, the last book of the Bible. In the twenty-eighth chapter of the book of Ezekiel in the Old Testament, the prophet, in vision, describes Lucifer, his elevated and anointed position in heaven and his spectacular fall from God's grace (Ezek. 28:12–19).

The devil or Satan lied about God's character, saying that He was not a loving God and did not care about us humans. In fact, Satan charged the Lord as being the sworn enemy of humankind. He portrayed God as overly stern, one to be feared, who forced His created heavenly beings (the angels) to do His bidding rather than His creation following and worshipping Him out of love. The devil charged that no one, given the choice, would serve God. Even if they did, they would fail because God's expectations were impossible to measure up to. Basically, it was at this point that the Lord decided to allow His character to be put on trial for the whole universe to see.

So then, the most amazing selfless act of love was put in place. God's Son Jesus came to earth as a human, lived a perfect life, and despite being completely innocent, died a horrible death by being crucified on a cross—a sacrificial death so that each one of us, by simply surrendering our hearts to Him, could live forever with Jesus in heaven.

But there's more to it than even that. What other reasons were there for Jesus to die a death reserved for only the most despicable and repugnant of criminals?

In Ken McFarland's excellent book, The Lucifer Files, he outlines very clearly the further compelling reasons why Jesus paid the ultimate sacrifice for you and me.

> *Jesus died to prove that Satan's charges against God's character were false.* For centuries, Satan had harped away on the idea that God did not care for human beings—that He was, in fact, the sworn enemy of mankind. But Calvary proved just how much God did care! On the cross it became clear that God loved His created beings more than His own life.

> *Jesus died to unmask Satan's real character before the universe.* When Satan put his own Creator on the cross and tortured and murdered Him, he destroyed whatever trace of sympathy that may have remained for his cause anywhere in the universe. His claims for the superiority of his self-centered approach to government were exposed for the lies they were.

> *Jesus died to reconcile us to the Father.* When the human race sinned, it became estranged from God—hostile toward Him. But in giving His Son to die on the cross, God took the initiative to heal the broken relationship—to reconcile us to Himself. See 2 Corinthians 5:19.

> And how does the cross bring reconciliation? As it begins to dawn on us what Christ really did for us there—how He took the ultimate consequences of all our sins—how He unhesitatingly threw away His own life that we might live—how He made it possible for us once more to stand before God as if we had never sinned—as we see this amazing outpouring of love, we lose all appetite for our foolish rebellion and return gladly to our Father's arms.

> *Jesus died as us.* And what does that mean? It means that just as we were all included in Adam when he sinned and therefore were doomed to reap the inevitable consequences of sin, just so through God we were also included in Christ—who reaped those deadly consequences for us. As the second Adam—the new head

of the human race—Christ is sinless and guiltless before God. And unless we refuse to permit God to include us in Christ, we too stand perfect before our Father. But only as we are *in Christ*.

Jesus died to prove that His law could not be changed. From the beginning of the great controversy, Satan had attacked God's eternal law. In heaven, as Lucifer, he had challenged God's law of love. And God's law, which is simply a perfect transcript of His own character of love, cannot be broken without penalty.

Once Lucifer himself broke God's law, he realized he would inevitably reap the natural consequence of his own rebellious choice—death. Therefore, he lobbied hard to persuade God to set aside His law in just this one case.

But God could not set aside His law without bringing in chaos. The whole foundation of happiness for the universe would crumble. Seeing that God would not set aside the law for him, Lucifer declared war on it, calling it unfair, arbitrary, and impossible to keep. And when Adam and Eve joined him in disobedience, this seemed to prove the devil's point that the law could not be kept.

If God could have set His law aside, or changed it, then no penalty or consequences would follow breaking it. And if no one needed to reap that penalty of death, Christ did not need to die on the cross. Christ's death on Calvary proved that the law could not be changed—that someone had to reap its inevitable consequences.

Jesus died to sin-proof the universe. Once this great controversy—this great experiment in rebellion—is over, sin will never rise up again. See Nahum 1:9. Why? Will God take away our free will? Will He program us like so many computers so that we have no choice but to worship Him and keep His law?

No, God has chosen instead to immunize us against sin. You see, Calvary proves to us once and for all that *sin kills*! Sin *always* kills. Death is its inescapable consequence. And as we see what happened to Jesus when He took the consequences of our own sins, we will come to hate sin with an ever-deepening passion. [2]

---

[2] K. McFarland, *The Lucifer Files* (Boise, ID: Pacific Press, 1988), p. 96–98.

From these six points, we clearly see that God and His character was completely vindicated when Jesus died for us on the cross.

For millennia, then, the inhabitants of earth have been caught up in the middle of a great controversy between Jesus Christ and Satan. The great controversy ends essentially when two things occur:

1. When sin, in all its horrible forms on this earth, has filled up the cup of God's wrath and is on the point of overflowing.

2. When as many people as possible will turn to God to be sealed and saved, then Jesus will return to earth in glory, resurrecting those who died in His name and claiming those righteous who are still living. They will all be taken up to heaven, the wicked will be destroyed, and Satan will be confined to the earth alone to contemplate his situation.

Without going into all the specifics, after 1,000 years, the New Jerusalem with all God's people will descend from heaven to the earth made new. Satan, his evil angels, and those who did not accept Christ before His return will be finally vanquished. In fact, Satan, along with those who have not given their hearts to the Lord, will come up in the final judgment and then, sadly, will lose out on eternal life—their lives will be permanently ended. (For all the details on this, read Revelation, the last book of the Bible.)

Now we know in truth that *Satan*, not God, is the enemy, the vilest offender and perpetrator of evil in this world. Although it is complicated, it is essentially Satan who is responsible for all the disease, pain, sickness, suffering, heartache, death, earthquakes, tornados, tsunamis, fires, etc.

One very excellent study vindicating God and exposing Satan for who he really is, is found in detail in the book of Job where we read the fascinating story of this wealthy man named Job. No matter what Satan tried to take away from him or inflict him with, Job would not turn away from God. In fact, his famous response to those who told him to "curse God, and die" (Job 2:9, KJV) was, "Though he slay me, yet will I trust in him" (Job 13:15, KJV). Now that is what I call trust in the Lord!

Yet another aspect of trusting in God is the issue of guilt and not feeling worthy of God's love. Having these guilt feelings makes it very difficult to have a healthy and satisfying relationship with God.

We may feel that we have committed certain things in our past that we are not too proud of. Surely the Lord would not want to have anything to do with us who have done what, in our mind, is unforgivable. Thankfully, nothing could be further from the truth! There are *no* unforgivable sins (unless we decide to reject the gift of accepting Jesus' Holy Spirit and His forgiveness, which is referred to in the Bible as the *unpardonable sin* [Matt. 12:31–32])!

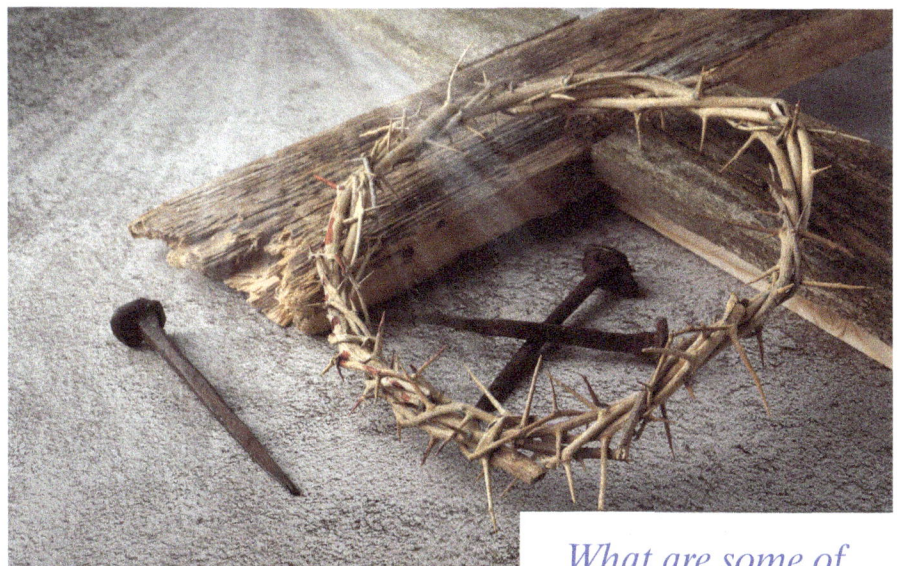

Jesus has paid the ultimate price for our sins by laying down His life so that we could live. He asks us to come to Him just as we are, to repent of our sin, and ask forgiveness. This is a promise that Jesus has made and as long as sin remains on this planet, His forgiveness remains and can never be taken away or changed.

What are some of the health benefits of having a living faith or trust in Jesus Christ? Well, there are many—too many, in fact, to list here but I will mention a few that may even surprise you.

> *What are some of the health benefits of having a living faith or trust in Jesus Christ? Well, there are many—too many, in fact, to list here but I will mention a few that may even surprise you.*

- *Reader's Digest* has reported that in a nationwide study of 21,000 people, those who prayed and attended religious services more than once a week had a seven-year longer life expectancy for

Caucasians and potentially fourteen years for African Americans than those who never attended services.[3]
- When we trust in the Lord we will grow and be *transformed* in all other areas of our lives: Rest, Activity, Nutrition, Supplementation, our Finances, Outlook, Relationships, and Motivation.
- As we internalize Christ's unconditional love for us, research shows, "Unconditional love is the most powerful stimulant of the immune system. The truth is love heals."[4]
- Feeling love for and feeling loved by God resulted in higher self-esteem, higher levels of self-efficacy or sense of mastery, less depression, less physical disability, greater self-rated health.[5]
- Frequent prayer, whether public or private, is associated with better health and emotional well-being and lower levels of psychological distress.[6]
- Several studies have found that people who rated themselves as more religious had greater life satisfaction[7], greater happiness, fewer symptoms of anxiety or depression, a more positive outlook, higher level of emotional balance[8], more meaningful relationships, and better health.
- A review of over sixty studies looked at the relationship between suicide and religion and found 84 percent lower rates of suicide (and more negative attitudes toward suicide) among the more religious.[9] This is especially significant since US suicide rates are at their highest since World War II, according to federal data.[10]
- Reviews of more than 1,200 published studies in physical, mental, and social health fields revealed that the majority of studies indicate that religiousness is associated with less coronary artery disease, hypertension, stroke, immune system dysfunction, cancer

---

[3] M. Musick, "Religion and Subjective Health Among Black and White Elders," *Journal of Health and Social Behaviour* 37 (1996): pp. 221–237.
[4] B. Siegel, *Love, Medicine & Miracles: Lessons Learned About Self-Healing from a Surgeon's Experience with Exceptional Patients* (New York, NY: Harper Perennial, 1986), p. 181.
[5] J. Levin, *God, Faith and Health: Exploring the Spirituality-Healing Connection* (New York, NY: John Wiley and Sons, Inc., 2001), p. 128.
[6] Ibid., p. 77
[7] J. Levin, L. Chatters, et al., "Religious Effects on Health Status and Life Satisfaction Among Black Americans," *Journal of Gerontology: Social Sciences* 50B (1995): pp. 154–163.
[8] J. Levin and C. Ellison, "Modeling Religious Effects on Health and Psychological Well-Being: A replicated Secondary Data Analysis of Seven Study Samples," Unpublished research quoted in J. Levin, *God, Faith and Health*, p. 131.
[9] H.G. Koenig, M. McCullough, and D.B. Larson, *Handbook of religion and health: a century of research reviewed* (New York, NY: Oxford University Press, 2001), p. 217.
[10] Jamie Ducharme, "U.S. Suicide Rates Are the Highest They've Been Since World War II," *TIME*, https://1ref.us/1qa (accessed October 28, 2021).

and functional impairment, fewer negative health behaviours (e.g., smoking, drug and alcohol abuse, risky sexual behaviours, and sedentary lifestyle), and lower overall mortality.[11]

To summarize, trusting in the Lord, demonstrated empirically over thousands of years and now scientifically by research, is a fundamental, key factor in all aspects of health—mental, emotional, social, spiritual, and physical wellness. There are four steps that can be implemented to grow your trust in God so that it is a well-entrenched habit in your daily life:

1. Bible Study—Start prayerfully reading the gospel of John in the New Testament or the Psalms and go from there. Memorize a new Bible promise each week and see how your trust in the Lord grows.

2. Prayer (talking to God)—Begin to pray each day by talking to God anytime, anywhere, in any way, about anything. Believe He will hear your prayers and that He will answer them according to His will for you. It is much more likely that it would be God's will for you to successfully get through a major surgery than it is to give you that Mercedes that you have had your eye on.

3. Meditation (God talks to you)—This is not to be confused with Eastern philosophy which often teaches a person to go into an altered state of consciousness by chanting or repeating a mantra or some such thing. It is simply allowing God to speak to you in a quiet setting away from interruptions or distractions.

I often meditate when I am driving or out for a walk, but it can literally be anytime or anywhere. I simply let my mind gravitate to the things that are top of mind for the day or what Jesus puts into my mind to contemplate. It may be some trivial item or it may be something of great and pressing importance to you in your life.

I invite the Lord to help me find answers by simply saying, "Lord, what would you have me do in this situation?" or "How do I deal with _____?" or "What is Your will for me in my life today?" Whatever it is that is on your mind, you have a Savior who is personally concerned with all your problems, worries, and challenges. He will help you to resolve your issues in His time as He sees fit.

Another way to meditate as a Christian is to open your Bible to a particular verse that you would like to read or just open the Word anywhere.

---

11   H.G. Koenig, "Religion, Spirituality and Health: The Research and Clinical Implications," *ISRN Psychiatry* (2012).

Read over the passage slowly two, three, or more times and then reflect or meditate on that Scripture. Keep your mind focused on what you have read, and jot down on paper what good thoughts and meaning you receive from these verses and how you can incorporate these thoughts into your life.

There are numerous wonderful benefits of Christian meditation. Here are some of the main ones.

    a) Your faith will increase because you are developing a stronger relationship with God. By getting to know Him and seeing how He graciously works out the big and the little things in your life, you begin to trust Him more and more as time goes on. This experience is golden, and it only gets better as you are faithful to this.

    b) Meditation is a wonderful hedge against sin in your life. You may be struggling with certain sins, perhaps overindulgence in appetite or alcohol or any other idol, as well as anger, immoral thoughts, jealousy, etc. Through meditation and prayer, you can give it over to the Lord and focus on Him and His goodness and mercy toward you. The Lord will empower you with the strength to overcome the temptations which may constantly be oppressing you. Some of our sins we may actually cherish but we know that they don't sit right with Jesus and are a snare which will sooner or later catch up with us.

So, you may be wondering what I mean when I talk about food or appetite as being an idol. Isn't an idol something you worship? As a Christian, idolatry connotes the worship of something or someone other than God as if it were God. Simply stated, modern idols represent something or someone that we love more than Jesus. We regard this as being more important or taking more precedence in our lives than God.

The Lord has expressly commanded us in the Bible in several places that He wants every part of us and that we are to hold Him supreme in our affections. For example, in Exodus in the giving of the Ten Commandments, the very first commandment states, "You must not have any other god but me. You must not make for yourself an idol of any kind or an image of anything in the heavens or on the earth or in the sea" (Exod. 20:3–4, NLT).

Now today in our modern world, for the most part, the majority of us are not bowing down to statues or praying to gods of wood or stone. However, there are many things (idols) that we can get caught up in such as social media, sports, a hobby, food, fashion, gambling, sex, entertainers, actors, music, television, movies ... the list goes on and on.

Apart from your job (for some that becomes their idol), an idol today is basically something that you are spending more time at than your devotion to Christ and your service to Him. This is something that we all must watch out for. It is a trap that Satan uses to draw us away from our relationship with the Lord and thereby stunts our spiritual growth. It may even sabotage our salvation. Along with prayer and enlisting the support of the Holy Spirit, meditating on the Lord is very powerful in overcoming these besetting sin problems.

    c) Your love for God will grow as you become more aware of all He has done and is continuing to do for you. You will start to see more clearly even the smallest blessings that come your way that you perhaps just took for granted before.

    d) As you meditate on the Lord, worry and stress will start to melt away. One very important aspect of trusting in the Lord is to take on an "attitude of gratitude." As we meditate on His goodness, lovingkindness, and unconditional love toward us, and respond with gratitude, it has been scientifically proven that we cannot be anxious and grateful at the same time.[12] Just keep thanking Him for His grace, and worry and stress will melt away. Isn't that wonderful?

    e) Your understanding of God and the meaning of the passages in the Bible will grow. So too will your understanding of the plan and purpose that the Lord has for you in your life.

6. Sharing your faith. This happens through family worship, service and spiritual guidance to your family and others, humanitarian/mission projects, getting involved in a faith community, and learning to give Bible studies.

Extra TRANSFORMational Tips for Trust in the Lord:

"In God We Trust" has been the official motto of the United States since 1956. "In God We Trust" first appeared on U.S. coins in 1864 and Congress passed a law that was approved by President Eisenhower on July 30, 1956, declaring "In God We Trust" must appear on all currency. It has been used on paper currency since 1957. Another interesting fact is that it

---

12 Madhuleena R. Chowdhury, "The Neuroscience of Gratitude and How It Affects Anxiety and Grief," *Positive Psychology*, https://1ref.us/1qb (accessed October 28, 2021).

is also the motto of the U.S. State of Florida and the Republic of Nicaragua.[13] According to a 2003 joint poll by USA Today CNN and Gallup, 90 percent of Americans support the inscription "In God We Trust" on U.S. coins![14]

The Christian faith is the only religion which has as its basic foundation, a God who is personal and cares about our every need. As we pointed out earlier, Jesus Christ claimed that as the Son of God, He was, in fact, one with God. The Bible clearly describes Jesus as the Creator, creating all things—including us. He came to earth to exonerate God's character as a loving God and to sacrifice His life as an offering in our place so that upon accepting Him, we sinful humans could live eternally with Him in heaven.

All this is to say that, knowing that a poll showing that 90 percent of Americans support "In God We Trust," and that when people are in dire straits or facing life-threatening crises, they typically turn to God, crying out for help, for deliverance, and for hope—why wait till then? You can trust in the Lord right now and in every situation.

Compared to viewing God as a distant, uncaring, cold, remote, unapproachable Supreme Being, "Intelligent Designer," "the Universe", or as a "Force," Jesus Christ has offered us a personal relationship with Him that is real and most rewarding.

Don't wait until that major crisis occurs or when you are on your deathbed taking your last breath, or worse, dying suddenly in a car crash or other natural disaster. At that point, it is too late.

Take the time now to pray to the Lord for forgiveness of all your sins and invite Jesus into your heart. It will be the best decision you will ever make—not to mention, it will greatly enhance your mental, physical, and spiritual health.

I can't imagine where I would be today had I not surrendered my heart to Jesus more than forty years ago! By experiencing a personal relationship with Jesus, you can enjoy the benefits of heaven on earth now and be assured of eternal life after you die!

---

13 New World Encyclopedia, "Nicaragua," https://1ref.us/1qc (accessed October 28, 2021).
14 Aaron Miller, "'In God We Trust' a motto or more?" The Clarion, https://1ref.us/1qd (accessed October 28, 2021).

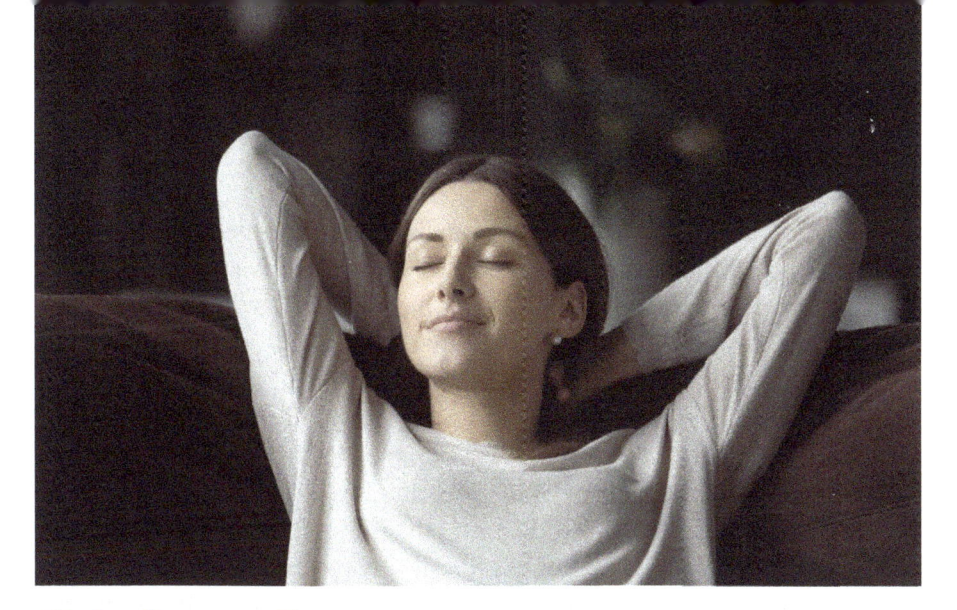

R is for … Rest

As we consider Rest as a part of TRANSFORMing our lives, it is important to look at it from different perspectives. We might think that getting a good sleep every night is all there is to rest, but it goes much further and deeper than that. If we consider the fact that chronic stress is linked to the six leading causes of death[15], rest and relaxation become of major and significant importance. While we need our daily rest and relaxation, we also need weekly, monthly, and annual rest to properly fulfill this most important health factor.

Let's break rest down into these four categories and explore the benefits of each.

Daily Rest: This means taking some time to relax or rejuvenate during the day. With our busy lives, many would say this is impossible, yet it can be done when you are intentional about it. For example, get up from your desk for a minute or two every half hour or less to change the environment, stretch, get a glass of water, or just walk around.

Practice taking deep breaths whenever you think about it, especially during your stretch breaks. Use part of your lunch hour to walk and be mobile. Make it your highest priority to get outside in the fresh air, even if it is only for a few minutes. Even though we may think outdoor air is worse than the air quality inside, the EPA states that the levels of indoor air pollutants are often two to five times higher than outdoor levels, and

---

15 Deborah S. Hartz-Seeley, "Chronic stress is linked to the six leading causes of death," *Miami Herald*, https://1ref.us/1qe (accessed October 28, 2021).

in some cases these levels can exceed 100 times that of outdoor levels of the same pollutants.[16]

I encourage a daily vacation where you spend some time thinking, meditating, or doing something you truly enjoy such as a hobby, a sport, or an activity like gardening, reading, or playing an instrument.

We also can't overlook the importance of getting a good rest each night. Sleep deprivation has become a huge problem in our Western world, leading to many health challenges and safety issues. Research underscores what I see in my clinic with a greater risk of obesity, cardiovascular disease, diabetes, hypertension, depression, and lowered immunity.

A University of Chicago study found that chronic sleep loss could hasten the onset, and increase the severity of diabetes, high blood pressure, and obesity.[17] Lack of sleep is also linked to a significantly increased risk of coronary heart disease.[18] Not enough sleep can also result in excessive daytime sleepiness, reduced neurocognitive function,[19] and depression.[20]

Research presented at the 1993 annual conference of the World Federation of Sleep Society reported that losing three hours of sleep on any given night can cut *in half* the effectiveness of an individual's immune system.[21] There is also evidence for a decrease in memory and learning.[22]

Be sure to get a minimum of seven to eight hours of good sleep each night. Surprisingly 30–40 percent of North Americans report less than six hours of sleep per night.[23]

If some sleep is good, more is better, right? Believe it or not, sleeping nine hours or more is actually *as harmful* health wise as getting six hours or less each night.

---

16   U.S. Environmental Protection Agency, 1987, "The total exposure assessment methodology (TEAM) study: Summary and analysis." https://1ref.us/1q4 (accessed August 26, 2021).
17   K. Spiegel et al., "Sleep curtailment in healthy young men is associated with decreased levels of leptin, elevated ghrelin levels, and increased hunger and appetite," *Annals of Internal Medicine* 141 (2004): pp. 846–850.
18   Najib Ayas et al., "A Prospective Study of Sleep Duration and Coronary Heart Disease in Women," *Journal Archives of Internal Medicine* 163 (2003): pp. 205–209.
19   Najib Ayas et al., "A Prospective Study of Self-Reported Sleep Duration and Incident Type 2 Diabetes in Women," *Diabetes Care* 26 (2003): pp. 380–384.
20   M. Patlak, U.S. Department of Health and Human Services, National Institutes of Health and National Heart, Lung and Blood Institute, "Your Guide to Healthy Sleep," NIH Publication No. 11-5271, November 2005. Revised August 2011.
21   James Perl, *Sleep Right in Five Nights: a clear and effective guide for conquering insomnia* (New York, NY: William Morrow and Company, Inc., 1993), p. 32.
22   Andrew J. Howell, Jesse C. Jährig, and Russell A. Powell, "Sleep quality, sleep propensity and academic performance," *Perceptual & Motor Skills*, October 2004.
23   Shawn Youngstedt et al., "Has Adult Sleep Duration Declined Over the Last 50+ Years?" NCBI, https://1ref.us/1qf (accessed October 28, 2021).

Researchers discovered that subjects who reported short (six or less hours per night) or long sleep (nine or more hours) shortened their lives by an average of *nine* years when compared with people who slept seven to eight hours per night.[24] Requiring that much sleep indicates that something is not quite right and should be checked out by a qualified health practitioner.

The question is often raised: What is the best time to go to bed? One important consideration for a restful sleep would be to retire at night when you feel most sleepy. This will vary as some people are "nighthawks" and others are "morning larks." Younger children tend to retire earlier in the evening, whereas high school and college-age individuals tend to retire later. After one reaches their thirties and beyond, the tendency is to retire earlier and earlier. Adjusting for these biological realities makes for healthier attitudes about ideal bedtimes.

Make sure your room is darkened *completely*, including all light emanating from windows, digital clocks, indicator lights, smartphones, etc. Keep all cellular technology and computers preferably in another room. If you must have your cellphone charging in your room, have it at least three feet away from your head to avoid radiation from EMF (electromagnetic fields). Better yet, put your phone on airplane mode or turn it off altogether.

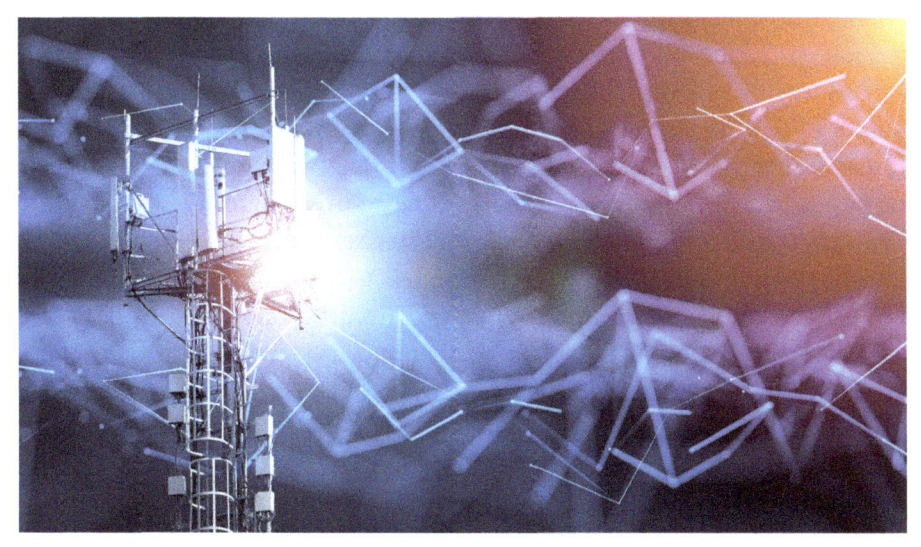

The radiation emitted from cell phones, cordless phones, computers, Wi-Fi, antennas, toasters, hair blowers, microwave ovens, electric baseboard heaters, flat-screen TVs, and other electronic appliances is called

---

24 Deborah Wingard and Lisa Berkman et al., "Mortality risk associated with sleeping patterns among adults," *Sleep* 6 (1983): pp. 102–107.

non-ionizing radiation. This form of electromagnetic radiation (EMR) or electromagnetic frequencies (EMF) causes thermal (heat-inducing) effects and can induce physiological health problems.

EMR is an ever-growing source of toxicity and stress to the body. Add on to that, EMR coming from microwave cellphone towers, radio frequencies (RF), etc. and you have a level of bombardment that, if visible through the human eye, would shock you. The bad news is, it will only become more significant as time goes on. 5G networks are now being introduced and 6G and beyond are in the works.

Research shows that EMFs from these devices can accumulate over time in your body. There has been a growing consensus in the scientific community that EMFs predominantly affect neurological tissue, and the largest collection of this tissue is the brain.

It is well-documented that cell phones, which emit electromagnetic fields in the radio frequency range, can cause DNA damage, headaches, blurred vision, dizziness, fatigue, short term memory loss, neuralgias, tumors, sleep disturbances, aberrant brain wave activity, and changes to cerebral blood flow, including altering the permeability of the blood brain barrier.[25]

Correlations have been shown between low fertility rates, low sperm count, and other reproductive issues when mobile smartphones are placed in close proximity to the testes, such as in a back pants pocket.[26] Having this source of radiation close to *any* tissue in the body for any extended length of time is tantamount to a ticking time bomb. With breast cancer rates as they are, I cringe when I see a young woman keep her phone tucked in her bra or in her back pocket close to the reproductive organs. With prostate and testicular cancer on the rise, men would be advised to avoid having an activated smartphone close to these areas.

These findings, both the association and dose relationships between cell phone usage and disease, place cell phone users into a high-risk health group. Children are even more vulnerable because of their developing brains and other organs.

Knowing that EMF effects are on a cumulative basis, recent studies have concluded that those who used cell phones for greater than ten

---

25 L. G. Salford et al., "Permeability of the blood-brain barrier induced by 915 MHz electromagnetic radiation, continuous wave and modulated at 8, 16, 50, and 200 Hz," *Microscopic Research Technology* 27 (1994): pp. 535-542.
26 Mohammed Abu El-Hamd and Soha Aboeldahab, "Cell phone and male infertility: An update," *Journal of Nephrology and Andrology*, https://1ref.us/1qg (accessed October 28, 2021).

years have a significantly increased risk of glioma, a form of brain tumor.[27] High-grade astrocytomas (aka. glioblastoma multiforme) are the most frequently occurring and most malignant glioma.

What can be done to protect against this invisible hazard to our health? We have become so dependent on our smartphones that we can hardly function without them. With no thanks to governments or the manufacturers themselves to be responsible for mitigating these very real risks, we turn to researchers, who on their own have come up with a solution. Enter Noise Field Technology or Molecular Resonance Effect Technology (MRET).

In the days of the Cold War, microwave radiation (all wireless communication is microwave radiation) was being used as a weapon. In a move to offset this threat, the U.S. Army funded a project that led to the discovery of the noise field. Litovitz discovered that when a random waveform was able to attach itself to a potentially damaging electromagnetic radiation wave, the new resultant wave caused no damage.[28]

Many others have corroborated the finding and thus there was really no reason to give up the benefits of our newfound communication advances if someone had the capability to develop a portable noise field. A scientist by the name of Igor Smirnov did exactly that, creating a Molecular Resonance Effect Technology that used ambient radiation to generate a noise field masking the damaging radiation and eliminating a physiological response.[29]

The science behind this discovery is substantial, showing the ability of cells to detect even very weak noise fields. It has been clearly proven that the MRET polymer chip generates a noise field and the **elimination** of electromagnetic radiation damage. The equation is simple: RADIATION + NOISE FIELD = NO PHYSIOLOGICAL EFFECTS.[30]

---

27 Nancy Wertheimer and Ed Leeper, "Adult cancer related to electrical wires near the home," *International Journal of Epidemiology* 11 (1982): pp. 345–355.
28 T. A. Litovitz et al., "Superimposing spatially coherent electromagnetic noise inhibits field-induced abnormalities in developing chick embryos," *Bioeletromagnetics* 15 1994: pp.105–113; T. A. Litovitz et al., "Bioeffects induced by exposure to microwaves are mitigated by superposition of ELF noise," *Bioelectromagnetics* 18 (1997): pp. 422–430; T. A. Litovitz, D. Krause, C. J. Montrose, and J. M. Mullins, "Temporally incoherent magnetic fields mitigate the response of biological systems to temporally coherent magnetic fields," *Bioelectromagnetics* 15 (1994): pp. 399–409.
29 Igor Smirnov, "Electromagnetic Radiation Optimum Neutralizer," *Explore Magazine* 11 (2002): pp. 45–50.
30 T. A. Litovitz et al., "Bioeffects induced by exposure to microwaves are mitigated by superposition of ELF noise," *Bioelectromagnetics* 18 (1997): pp. 422–430.

A study was conducted to examine the effects of cell phone radiation on normal human astrocytes and the effects of mobile phone radiation on normal human astrocytes when the MRET-Nylon polymer was used as an intervention to radio frequency radiation of the mobile phone.

The results demonstrated that the mobile phone radiation decreased the number of normal human astrocytes and when the cell phone was used with the intervention of the MRET-Nylon polymer, the number of normal human astrocytes increased.[31]

The wonderful news from all this is that the purchase of a small polymer chip can be applied to your smartphone, in your car, at your computer desk, on your computer, the headboard of your bed, anywhere you have a significant degree of EMFs that are being emitted. The chip will confer protection from EMFs within a radius of two meters in all directions from where it is applied.

Spending time on the computer or your smartphone is not a "smart" idea either. According to research, the blue light emitted from these screens has a detrimental effect on your brain which seems to get confused with the brightness of the screen, and this in turn upsets the brain's 24-hour circadian rhythm.[32]

Blue light eyeglasses have emerged, its makers claiming that it will block blue light, decrease eyestrain, improve sleep, prevent eye disease, and increase melatonin nighttime levels by about 58 percent.[33] Organizations like the American Academy of Ophthalmology dispute these benefits and say they don't really work and aren't necessary.[34] There is a lack of credible research at

> *Before retiring for the night, read something pleasant and practice gratitude. Think of three things that happened over the day that you can thank Jesus for. Many times, I am already asleep before I even get to the third one.*

---

31   Igor V. Smirnov, "The Exposure of Normal Human Astrocytes Cells to Mobile Phone Radiation with and without MRET-Nylon Protection," *European Journal of Scientific Research* 37 (2009): pp. 219–225.
32   Harvard Health Letter, "Blue Light Has a Dark Side," *Harvard Health Publishing*, https://1ref.us/1qh (accessed October 28, 2021).
33   Ralph Ellis, "Pandemic Screen Time: Will Blue Light Glasses Help?" WebMD, https://1ref.us/1qi (accessed October 28, 2021).
34   Ibid.

this time, but many insist that it has helped them, so ... try it if you like and see what you find.

Before retiring for the night, read something pleasant and practice gratitude. Think of three things that happened over the day that you can thank Jesus for. Many times, I am already asleep before I even get to the third one.

There are many other tips and strategies for a good night's rest, some which are helpful, some which are not. It is important to avoid eating your dinner or a snack too close to bedtime. This will disturb your sleep and your digestion both as they will conflict with one another the entire night.

Avoid sleep-depriving substances such as alcohol, caffeine, nicotine, etc., which interfere with the body's ability to get into the deeper, most restful stages of sleep as well as the all-important REM (rapid eye movement) stage. For obvious reasons, watching the late evening news or settling down to a horror movie or anything else that may cause anxiety should not be become a bedtime habit either.

Another disruptor of sleep which is becoming more understood, and as a result more diagnosed, is Obstructive Sleep Apnea (OSA). Essentially, it is a sleep-related breathing disorder that involves a decrease or complete halt in airflow despite an ongoing effort to breathe. It occurs when the muscles relax during sleep, causing soft tissue in the back of the throat to collapse and block the upper airway.

According to the American Academy of Sleep Medicine (AASM), about 80 to 90 percent of adults with OSA remain undiagnosed.[35] If a person snores loudly and frequently, with periods of silence when airflow is reduced or blocked, that is a red flag. Typically, they will then make choking, snorting, or gasping sounds when their airway reopens.

Although there are a number of risk groups, those who are at the most risk are those who are overweight or obese. For many, losing weight will correct the condition.

Occurrence is more frequent in men with 24 percent as compared to 9 percent in women.[36] It occurs most often between middle and older age groups. There are three different types: mild, moderate, and severe. In severe OSA, you can actually stop breathing more than thirty times per hour!

Besides being greatly disruptive to good quality sleep, the possible disturbing effects of OSA are numerous.

---

35 American Academy of Sleep Medicine, "Obstructive Sleep Apnea," https://1ref.us/1qj (accessed October 28, 2021).
36 Ibid

One major problem is daytime sleepiness which may affect your work performance (e.g., falling asleep while working or during meetings), your concentration, mood, and even an increased risk of being involved in a deadly motor vehicle accident.

Troubling as these possibilities may be, the most pressing concern, however, is OSA's effect on cardiovascular health. Typical symptoms are fluctuating oxygen levels, increased heart rate, and chronic elevation in daytime blood pressure. Most worrisome is increased risk of stroke and higher rate of death due to heart disease.[37]

OSA also ties into diabetes risk with impaired glucose tolerance and insulin resistance.[38]

If you or your spouse are experiencing disrupted sleep and your situation is similar to what I have described above, see your doctor to get a referral for a sleep study. If you are diagnosed with OSA, this may be one of the single most important steps you will have made to prevent one or more of the abovementioned health risks. There are various treatment options that, *if followed*, are quite effective in relieving this condition.

Of course, the other spouse/partner of a snorer often suffers from poor, interrupted sleep as well. If your partner is dragging their feet at getting it checked out, don't just put up with it and undermine your own well-being. Lovingly suggest that you both need separate rooms to solve your sleep challenges.

A word on sleep aids—I typically advise to steer clear of over-the-counter (OTC) and prescription drugs for sleep. Work really hard to determine what the source of your insomnia is and take measures to correct that cause. Because the origin(s) can be tricky at times to accurately assess, I recommend seeing a qualified natural health practitioner who is experienced with this and who will take the time to assist you with sorting this out. In addition to lifestyle changes, there are many good, safe, and non-addictive natural remedies that can help, depending on the root cause of the problem.

Weekly Rest: Did you know that God has given us fifty-two extra days off each year? It's true. If we look at the Fourth Commandment, it reads:

> Remember the Sabbath day, to keep it holy. Six days you shall labor and do all your work, but the seventh day *is* the Sabbath of the LORD your God. *In it* you shall do no work: you, nor your son, nor your daughter, nor your male servant, nor your female ser-

---

37 Ibid.
38 Ibid.

vant, nor your cattle, nor your stranger who *is* within your gates. For *in* six days the LORD made the heavens and the earth, the sea, and all that *is* in them, and rested the seventh day. Therefore, the LORD blessed the Sabbath day and hallowed it. (Exod. 20:8–11)

As we analyze this seventh day of the week that the Lord has not asked but commanded us to set apart, we see that if we are obedient to Him and abide by this rest day, we will receive not only spiritual rest and rejuvenation but mental and physical rest as well.

Our gracious and loving Lord Jesus, who created us, knows exactly what our needs are and has built in our makeup an internal, biological seven-day cycle—a seemingly endogenous rhythm that researchers have found called the circaseptan rhythm or seven-day period.[39]

Many think that it doesn't matter what day of the week you rest and worship God, but the Bible is very specific about it being the seventh day—Saturday and not Sunday or Friday or …. If you disagree, thinking that you are sure the Bible clearly says that we are to worship the Lord on Sunday, I challenge you to study your Bible and prove it. I humbly submit to you that you will not find a single verse in the Old or New Testament that commands us to worship God on Sunday.

In the book of Ezekiel 20 verses 19 and 20, the Lord declares: "I am the Lord your God; follow my decrees and be careful to keep my laws. Keep my Sabbaths holy, that they may be a sign between us. Then you will know that I am the Lord your God" (NIV). We see here that the Sabbath is a sign of obedience between us, His creation, and Him. In fact, God instituted the Sabbath at Creation (Gen. 2:1–3), and the Sabbath was even kept by God's people before Moses was presented with the Ten Commandments at Mount Sinai (Exod. 16:23–30). In the New Testament, we see that Jesus kept the Sabbath (Luke 4:16). His disciples kept it before Jesus was crucified and after He was resurrected (Acts 18:1–5). And in the book of Hebrews, it says: "For He has spoken in a certain place of the seventh day in this way: "And God rested on the seventh day from all His works." There remains therefore a rest for the people of God" (Heb. 4:4–9).

Added to that, God hallowed or sanctified that day *and that day only* as being holy. He knows that without specific guidance we as humans will find all kinds of different ways and days to rest or disregard rest altogether.

---

39 F. Levi and F. Halberg, "Circaseptan (about-7-day) bioperiodicity—spontaneous and reactive—and the search for pacemakers," Ric Clin Lab 12 (1982): pp. 323–370.

I am so thankful for this special day each week that the Lord has placed His stamp of approval on, where I can come apart from the daily activities of a busy, hectic week. I can have more meaningful time to grow closer not only to Jesus but also to my wife, family, and friends.

We often use this opportunity to get out in the fresh air and enjoy God's creation. Having that rest day rejuvenates me physically, calms the heart, reduces stress, anxiety, tension, and refreshes me before I dive back into the next week's active schedule.

A couple I know shared with me how much of an improvement having that rest day each week makes in their relationship. If they don't have that opportunity and miss that day together, their relationship suffers, and they find that they are more easily irritated and angry with each other. Having that day off to relax and enjoy each other's company makes a world of difference as they go through the new week.

From a health standpoint, those who keep the Sabbath day as part of a healthy lifestyle have been shown to enjoy greater health and longevity, to experience only a fraction of the diseases suffered by the average population and have a happier, more fulfilling life. It has led Dan Buettner, author of *The Blue Zones* to declare Seventh-day Adventists living around the Loma Linda area in California to be one of the *five longest living people groups in the world*.[40]

Monthly and Annual Rest can be dealt with together as they are simply more extended times of rest such as a weekend getaway, or a two or more weeks' vacation one or more times a year. It astounds me the number of patients that I see in my clinic that admit that they have not had a vacation in years!

My first counsel to them is to change that practice immediately. My reply to the response, "But, Doctor, I can't afford to take a holiday," is, "You can't afford *not* to take a holiday, even if it is just a day trip or a weekend here and there."

The most ideal vacation is to take two weeks or more at a given time to achieve the most complete and therapeutic opportunity to unwind and reset yourself mentally, emotionally, physically, and spiritually.

A true vacation should be taken away from home, unplugged from technology and where you can truly rest and relax, doing primarily the things that you enjoy doing and perhaps don't get a chance to do the rest of the year.

---

[40] Jamie Ducharme, "5 Places Where People Live the Longest and Healthiest Lives," February 15, 2018, https://1ref.us/1qk (accessed October 28, 2021).

Extra TRANSFORMational Tips for Rest:
- Make sure you have a good and comfortable mattress.
- Sleep in a room that is slightly cool rather than warm.
- Take an Epsom salt bath and add relaxing essential oils to the bath water.
- Use an aromatherapy diffuser and add in single or blended essential oils that are specific for sleep and relaxation.
- Use foam earplugs and eye covers if needed.
- • Massage therapy is often very helpful to improve sleep and help one unwind.
- • • If you are not sleeping through the night, perhaps having to get up one or more times through the night to void, try this simple but amazing strategy with melatonin. Melatonin is safe and easy to buy at any health food store and comes in different milligram (mg) strengths.

Start with 2 or 3 mg at bedtime to sleep more restfully with less or no interrupted sleep. Increase dose by 1–2 mg each night until you are sleeping right through the entire night. Your "dose" will vary from individual to individual and can go up as high as 25 mg or more. You can take your "dose" indefinitely to sleep well.
- • • • Many claim that taking 2,000 mg of vitamin C at bedtime really helps them with insomnia.

The Sabbath Day of Rest and the "Mark of the Beast"

Today, there is a sense that this planet is on a collision course with destiny. Many believe we are living in the last days of earth as we know it, heading toward some sort of cataclysmic conflict—Armageddon, if you like.

A careful study of the last book in the Bible called the Revelation to Saint John the Divine or also known as the apocalypse shows that obedience to the seventh day of worship and rest that God ordained and never changed, will figure in to the *mark of the beast and the seal of God* mentioned in this most fascinating, prophetic book.

Let's examine what a seal represents. If we use the seal of the president of the United States as an example, it identifies the name or the responsibility of the person—in this case, the president. It represents the jurisdiction over which he has his authority—the United States.

The seal of God then identifies God as our Creator, who is God of the universe (Gen. 1:1), which includes us on planet earth. Behind the seal lies

His authority, which are His law and precepts which form the foundation of His eternal kingdom.

If someone were to receive the seal of God then, it would mean that they first have accepted Jesus Christ as God's Son, who died for us as sinners, paying the price for our sin by accepting one of the most abhorrent and heinous forms of cruelty—death by crucifixion. This realization and acceptance of what Jesus did for us leads us to love Him and to seek His forgiveness for our sins. We recognize the Lord as our supreme authority and are happily obedient to Him by being faithful in following all the Lord's laws (commandments) and principles.

The seal of God is received on the foreheads of those who are God's servants (Rev.7:2–17). Rather than a literal mark on the forehead, this signifies an intellectual assent or agreement. Contrast this with the *mark of the beast* which seeks to impose its authority by force. We see in Revelation chapter 13 that this huge beast received its power from the dragon who is identified as the devil or Satan (Rev.12:1–9). As it says in Revelation 13, this huge beast made all sorts of religious claims for itself and even blasphemed God by claiming to speak for God (Rev.13:5–8). It even persecuted and murdered millions upon millions of God's true followers through the centuries as it exacted its rule by forcing its doctrines upon the populace.

In verse 11 of Revelation 13, we see a lamblike animal emerging that eventually changes from a lamb into a dragon and begins to speak and act like one. This lamblike animal-turned-dragon becomes interested in the huge beast and the dragon who is Satan.

An image of the huge beast was set up by the animal who was given power to perform miracles by Satan (the dragon). The huge beast had suffered an almost fatal wound but managed to heal and received its power back. The animal had the power to breathe life into the image of the huge beast and soon there was a worldwide decree that threatened anyone with death who did not accept and worship the image of the huge beast. Everyone was forced to accept the mark of the huge beast in their right hands (by doing what it told them to do) or in their foreheads (by acknowledging its authority). No one could buy or sell anything unless they could prove their loyalty to the huge beast by having either the huge beast's mark or its number. Chapter 13 finishes by giving the number of the huge beast which is 666. It is the *number of a man*, not a creature (Rev. 13:18).

Whew! Seems rather complicated and confusing with all these dragons and beasts, doesn't it? Very simply stated, we know that this trilateral force which opposes the Trinity of God, His Son Jesus, and the Holy

Spirit consists of the dragon (Satan), the huge beast, and the lamblike-animal-turned-dragon. The huge beast represents a dominant religiopolitical power operating throughout the centuries and even right up to the present day. The animal represents a country which is a superpower today. Jesus said in Matthew 13:16 (ESV): "But blessed are your eyes, for they see, and your ears, for they hear."

Revelation is telling us that the *mark of the beast* is something that opposes the worship, the law, and the authority of God. No sooner does the huge beast regain power from its deadly wound, but it begins to persecute the saints (the Lord's true followers) again, thinking to change God's laws and forcing obedience to these changes. This huge beast has claimed, by its authority, that it changed the day of worship from Saturday to Sunday.

Revelation 14:1 tells us that those who refuse to accept the mark of the beast are *sealed in their foreheads* with the Father's name because they have accepted His authority above all others. I would submit to you that this very Sabbath day of rest which is the fourth commandment of the Ten Commandments is at the heart of the huge beast's persecution and his mark. From my years of study, I believe that the *mark of the beast will be about allegiance to authority—allegiance to the authority of the state (government) or allegiance to God. I believe the authority of God will be challenged by the state making a decree that Sunday must be kept sacred through a Sunday law.* All who agree with this deviation from the true Sabbath, or seventh day, will receive the *"mark."* Those who refuse to accept this Sunday law, and remain true to God and His long-established Sabbath day of worship, will receive the seal of God. Anyone refusing to keep the Sunday law will experience milder penalties and restricted freedoms at first. As times goes on, they will become harsher with the removal of the ability to buy or sell and eventually it will come to the death penalty itself.[41]

Please know that those who remain faithful to God and refuse to stop keeping the Sabbath will be under the Lord's protection despite what man may try to do. What a truly wonderful God we serve!

---

41 Revelation 13:11–18.

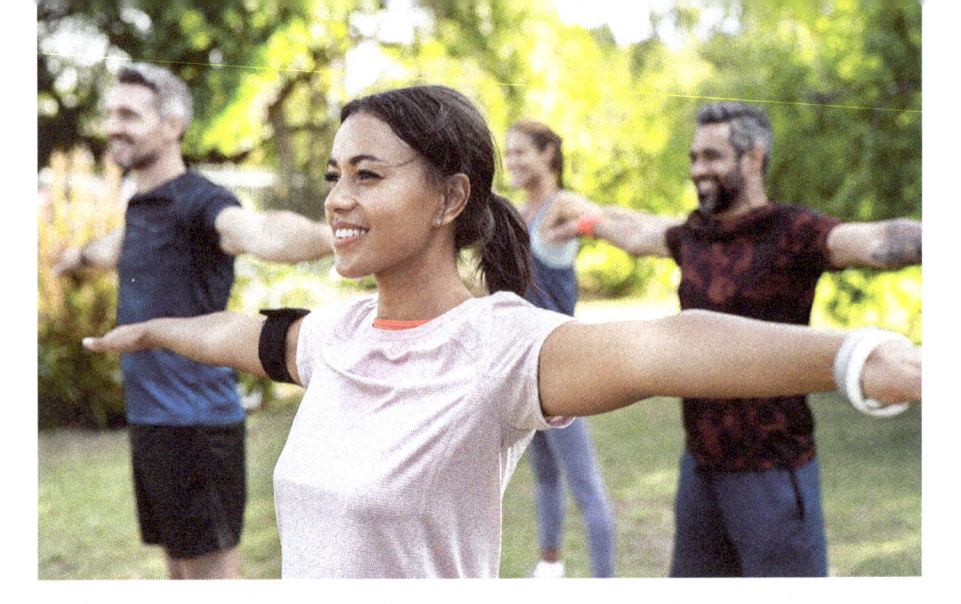

A is for ... Activity

We have chosen the word **activity** to represent not only the importance of physical activity but mental activity as well. When it comes to exercise, activity for most people is a far more "friendly" word than exercise. It conveys the idea that we can get our daily exercise by doing things that we *enjoy* rather than forcing ourselves to do something that we consider drudgery.

Physical Activity

I believe that God created us to be active—to be mobile and on the move. In fact, we find that in the beginning "the LORD God took the man and put him in the garden of Eden to tend and keep it" (Gen. 2:15). Those of you who do gardening and yard work know what a tremendous all-around activity this is for the body.

According to the mantra of the day, "sitting is the new smoking," living a sedentary lifestyle is deadly ... yet many people struggle to break out of this trap.

If you are prone to sitting a lot, either at home or at work, set your timer on your smartphone or stovetop or get an inexpensive timer from the dollar store and set it for thirty minutes. When it goes off, it is your signal to get up and move around, stretch, take a bio-break, have a glass of water, etc. This way, you ensure that you are not sitting for too long a stretch.

If you are watching TV, get up during the commercials and do something. If you are streaming and there are no commercials, pause it and take a few minutes break every half hour or so. You will see that it really makes a difference. You won't feel so sluggish or stiff after sitting in one place so long.

The key is, find an activity or activities that you enjoy and *get started* even if it is just a few minutes a day. Getting a membership at a gym is very beneficial, but it's not for everybody.

For me, it works because I need to physically get away from my office or home and go to a place where I can dedicate myself to exercise without interruptions. There is a lot of variety with all the different types of exercise equipment which helps to keep it interesting. Thankfully, for those who feel that a gym is the last place they want to be seen, there are many other options to get and keep physically fit. You can go hike, run, walk, swim, cycle, play a sport, garden, do work around the house—anything that you enjoy that keeps you physically active.

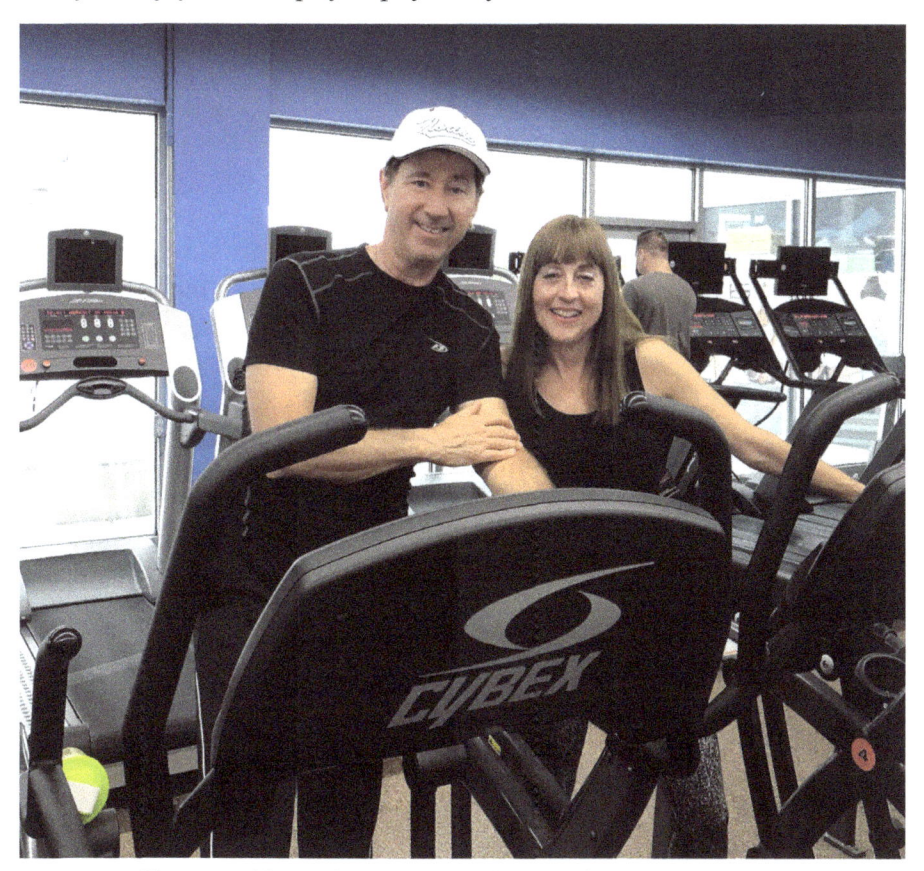

Dr. Sloan and his wife, Erika, on their 42nd wedding anniversary

Walking is One of the World's Best Kept Secrets

I recommend that in the absence of anything else, a person cannot go wrong with starting up a simple walking program. Research shows that despite the widespread indication that you must go to a gym to pump iron, get on the exercise machines and run ad nauseam on the treadmill for at least thirty minutes or more, a good walking program will accomplish much more than what was once thought. In fact, research has shown the following:

- Walking lowers body mass index (BMI)—an indicator of obesity.[42]
- Lowers blood pressure and cholesterol, with a "7 percent reduced risk of high blood pressure and high cholesterol."[43]
- Lowers fasting blood sugar—"the National Walkers' Health Study also found that walkers had a 12 percent lower risk of type 2 diabetes."[44]
- Better memory and cognitive function—"a study of 299 adults, published in the journal Neurology in 2010, found that walking was associated with a greater volume of gray matter in the brain, a measure of brain health."[45]
- Lower stress and improved mood. "[W]alking—especially out in nature—stimulates the production of neurotransmitters in the brain (such as endorphins) that help improve your mental state."[46]
- Longer life—roughly three hours a week of walking "was associated with an 11 percent reduced risk of premature death compared with those who did little or no activity."[47]

So, don't worry that you haven't got time or that you can't afford expensive gyms. Just simply get out and walk.

Getting **outside** to walk is *most* desirable because we need to get out from indoor pollution and breathe in *deeply* and freely of the fresh outside air.

---

[42] Sally Wadyka, "How to Get the Biggest Benefits of Walking," *Consumer Reports*, https://1ref.us/1ql (accessed October 28, 2021).
[43] Ibid.
[44] Ibid.
[45] Ibid.
[46] Ibid.
[47] Ibid.

Deep Breathing is of Vital Importance

Now, when I say deeply, I am deliberate in saying so. Most of us are shallow breathers. If you look into this, you will discover that it is true. Typically, we fill only one-third or less of our lungs when we breathe, so when you are walking, utilize this simple "seven-step" system that I use which works very well. I recommend starting with the **basic** form and work toward the advanced. Breathe in *as deep as you can through the nose* for four steps, and forcefully exhale, emptying your lungs completely through the mouth for steps five, six, and seven. Keep repeating this for at least five to ten times to start, making sure you are not feeling weak, light-headed, or dizzy.

Once you have this where you feel completely comfortable, you are ready to go ahead with the **advanced** form. Breathe in deeply again, fully expanding your lungs for the first four steps. Hold your breath for steps five, six, and seven, and *exhale as forcefully through the mouth as you can* while you walk the next seven steps. Inhale again for four steps, hold for three, then exhale again for the next seven. Each time you exhale, try to empty your lungs completely so there is barely any air left before inhaling again on step one. Continue to do this during a portion of your walk, or the entire time if you wish. Start with perhaps ten of these in succession and gradually work up to a minimum of twenty times or more during your walk.

One additional strategy is to walk up a steep embankment or you break into a run for a portion of your walk. Now, because of the increased need for oxygen as you have stepped things up, you can *breathe in for steps one, two, and three* and exhale steps *four through seven*. This allows you to get more air in quickly for times such as these.

Another interesting benefit from deep breathing is that it will support your immune system in its efforts to protect you.

A health secret that I have told numerous patients over the years is that if you feel like you are coming down with a sniffle, a cold, or some other "bug" of any sort, follow the abovementioned plan to do deep breathing while you are out walking in the fresh air. Bacteria, viruses, and other pathogens cannot survive in the presence of oxygen, so you are, in essence, targeting pathogens in an amazingly simple, inexpensive, and effective way!

Filling your lungs with fresh oxygen will go directly into the bloodstream and kill any pathogens present. Thus, you can use this approach to treat or prevent these common annoyances and get your exercise at the same time. For many people, if they catch it early enough, this may be all they need to stop it dead in its tracks. It is a total win-win situation, and it works.

In the beginning, all that oxygen being brought into the lungs could make some individuals a bit light-headed or dizzy, causing one to perhaps be unsteady or even faint. Exercise caution for the first while until you become accustomed to it. This very fact shows that you are not used to having optimal levels of oxygen in your system. The more you do this, the better you will feel and the more stamina you will experience.

At the same time, moderate exposure to sunlight is very beneficial to health and well-being in numerous ways, including eye health, vitamin D production, immune support, and mood enhancement.

Some years ago, John N. Ott published an excellent book entitled *Health and Light*. Amongst many other interesting facts about the importance of sunlight was the fact that our eyes need light—and specifically *sunlight*—for our health. The light from the sun, which is natural full-spectrum light, is taken in through our eyes and into the brain where it stimulates many health-promoting reactions that are conducive to better health. In fact, John Ott's book was a scientific exploration of numerous subjects involving light and human health including showing the health benefits of groups getting some daylight as opposed to those who prevented natural light coming in by wearing sunglasses, regular glasses, and contact lenses.[48]

We know now that vitamin D is a crucial nutrient which is important for a long list of important benefits in the body (more on this in the "S is for Supplementation" chapter). Getting sunlight is the way our bodies naturally produce vitamin D.

All we need is ten to thirty minutes of midday sunlight on as little as a few square inches of exposed skin several times per week. People with darker skin may need a little more than this. Your exposure time should depend on how sensitive your skin is to sunlight.[49]

The problem is most all of us who live in the more northern United States and Canada don't get enough sunlight and unless we take it in a supplementary form, we will be deficient in this vital nutrient. In fact, I have found in my own practice that patients who live in the regions mentioned above, who do not take a supplement of vitamin D3, are deficient almost 100 percent of the time when tested. This has been backed up in my own clinics with vitamin D testing.

---

48   John Nash Ott, *Health and Light* (New York, NY: Pocket Books, 2000).
49   Ryan Raman, "How to Safely Get Vitamin D From Sunlight," healthline, https://1ref.us/1qm (accessed October 28, 2021).

Walking is one of the most effective forms of exercise for the following reasons:

- almost anyone can walk
- it works the largest muscles of the body
- promotes cardiorespiratory endurance
- firms, strengthens, and tones the muscles, tendons, and ligaments
- promotes oxygenation to the heart, brain, blood, and muscles
- promotes calcium assimilation and utilization for bone development and stability
- is "low-impact" meaning less wear and tear on the joints
- is a great mental, physical, and emotional "stress-buster"
- can be done with a partner making it a social, fun activity
- reasonably inexpensive—a comfortable, but good quality, pair of shoes will do

If you are walking alone, make it interesting. There are a number of things you can do while walking, which is only limited by your creativity. You can listen to music, a podcast, an audiobook, a presentation, a lecture, or a seminar. Of course, if you are carrying a device like a smartphone, you will want to be sure that you have your noise field technology protective chip attached to your phone. (See chapter on Rest.)

You can pray, you can pray-walk (as you walk by each home, ask the Lord to place a special blessing on the occupants of the home and to minister to any special needs they may be having at that particular time).

You can prepare a speech, think about your day, warm up your voice if you are a singer or speaker, and anything else you might think of to do. At the very least you can enjoy the beautiful outdoors and experience nature as God intended.

Start at your own pace and go from there. Be careful not to overdo it or any other exercise program for that matter, especially if you have not been exercising for a while. If possible, try to walk on grass or a natural trail that is not paved. This is much less stressful on the joints of the body, reducing wear and tear.

As discussed above, because of the importance of unimpeded natural light for the eyes and vitamin D production by direct exposure of the sun on the skin, try to walk *without* sunglasses or sunscreen. Walking in the earlier part of the day, late afternoon, or early evening is more desirable from this aspect, but anytime of the day is good. And as mentioned earlier, good footwear is very important and not something you should "cheap out" on. But even further, if you are in a place where you can, walk barefoot.

Go Barefoot

Walking barefoot, which is also known as "earthing" or "grounding," may seem to be a "kooky" counterculture thing that dates back to the hippie movement of the sixties. Turns out that "earthing," along with a number of other ideas the hippies promoted, are now grounded in science. In a society which promotes the importance of wearing shoes continually, going barefoot is hardly popular, but you may think differently after you read about its proven benefits.

"According to Dr. Mercola, walking with your feet directly touching the soil allows your body to absorb negative electrons through the Earth, which helps to stabilize daily cortisol rhythm and create a balanced internal bioelectrical environment."[50]

The following are some of the important benefits that you may enjoy going barefoot.

1. Walking Barefoot Can Reduce Pain and Inflammation

A study[51] was done to see if sleeping on a mattress pad that mimicked the effect of sleeping directly on the earth would help with pain, stress, and trouble sleeping. Twelve people who had these symptoms were observed as they slept on this grounded mattress for eight weeks straight. Not only were their cortisol levels (a hormone associated with stress in the body) significantly lower, but they all reported that their pain, stress, and sleep troubles had either been greatly reduced or disappeared entirely. By walking barefoot, one is essentially doing the same thing by grounding your body to the earth.

2. It Can Help Improve Your Sleep

Another study in PubMed revealed that earthing influences physiologic processes and induces relaxation.[52] The Journal of Alternative and Complementary Medicine also reported that people who had been exposed to grounding had a better night's sleep compared with those who

---

50   "10 Surprising Health Benefits of Walking Barefoot," Power of Positivity, https://1ref.us/1qn (accessed October 28, 2021).
51   Maurice Ghaly and Dale Teplitz, "The biologic effects of grounding the human body during sleep as measured by cortisol levels and subjective reporting of sleep, pain and stress," *Journal of Alternative and Complementary Medicine* 10 (2004): pp. 767–776.
52   Karol Sokal and Pawel Sokal, "Earthing the human body influences physiologic processes," NCBI, https://1ref.us/1qo (accessed October 28, 2021).

did not walk barefoot regularly. Because earthing may stabilize circadian rhythms, this perhaps is why many people experience a better night's sleep.[53]

3. Walking Barefoot Helps Build the Immune System

In this comprehensive report[54] published in the Journal of Environmental and Public Health, researchers found that walking barefoot can actually decrease white blood cell count and increase red blood cell count. This outcome indicates a positive immune response.

4. Walking Barefoot Helps to Decrease Feelings of Anxiety and Stress

Getting outside is marvelous for helping to regulate emotions and balance the nervous system. However, when your feet come in contact with the soil directly, it can decrease anxiety and stress even more. This is due to the earth carrying a negative charge with it. With all the positive charge building up from daily bombardment with electromagnetic frequencies from microwave ovens, your hair blower, your smartphone, etc., spending time connecting with the earth is vital to your emotional and physical health.

5. It Helps Normalize Biological Rhythms

In the book *Earthing* by Clint Ober, Dr. Stephen Sinatra, and Martin Zucker, the authors explain that "[T]he biological clock of the body needs to be continually calibrated by the pulse of the Earth that governs the circadian rhythms of all life on the planet."[55]

"Earthing helps to re-establish regular sleeping patterns and resets the biological clock within us all. Environmental pollution, including lights, chemicals, and other factors, greatly affects our sleeping patterns, so coming in contact with Earth's negatively charged electrons can help immensely with your body's circadian rhythm and other biological processes."[56]

---

53 "10 benefits of walking with barefoot," https://1ref.us/1qp (accessed October 28, 2021).
54 Gaetan Chevalier, Stephen T. Sinatra and Pawel Sokal, "Earthing: Health Implications of Reconnecting the Human Body to the Earth's Surface Electrons," *Journal of Environmental and Public Health* (2012).
55 Clinton Ober, Stephen T. Sinatra and Martin Zucker, "Earthing: The Most Important Health Discovery Ever?" Basic Health Publications (2010): p.17.
56 Julia Kuburi, "9 Surprising Health Benefits of Walking Barefoot," *Medium*, https://1ref.us/1qq (accessed October 28, 2021).

6. Walking Barefoot Helps Loosen Tense Muscles, Eliminate Headaches, and Boost Energy Levels.

"A pilot study found that going barefoot can prevent delayed onset muscle soreness from occurring after engaging in physical exercise."[57] It may very likely apply to other situations that cause tense muscles, such as working at a desk all day, for example.

As far as energy levels go, whenever you are walking outside—especially barefoot—you pick up on the higher frequencies emitted from nature and thereby improve your energy levels.[58] Being indoors for extended periods of time and exposure to modern-day stresses and strains can definitely affect your vitality. So, get out and enjoy nature as much as you can … barefoot if possible. (For more information on the incredible ways that walking barefoot can improve your health, consider reading the book *Earthing: The Most Important Health Discovery Ever!* In it, you will find studies and other information from doctors, an electrical engineer, and a cardiologist. Also, you will find firsthand stories about the benefits of earthing.)

As you begin your walking program, gradually pick up the pace and try to walk just a bit further and longer each day until you are doing a minimum of thirty minutes three to five times or more per week. In no time, you will be strutting along with the best of them!

It is ideal to walk in the early morning or evening before sundown. Avoid wearing sunglasses to get the benefits of natural light, go barefoot if possible, deep breathe, and avoid using sunscreen which blocks vitamin D production.

When considering optimal physical activity, it is important to make sure that you include the three main forms of exercise:

1. Cardiovascular or aerobic exercise affords wonderful prevention for strokes, heart attacks, vascular disease, diabetes, etc. There is a vast amount of information on this subject depending on how deeply or intensively you want to delve into it. Suffice to say, when it helps to prevent coronary heart disease (CHD) which affects one in every two persons, it should be an important consideration in everybody's lifestyle plan. In addition to preventing CHD, it has a favorable effect on the prevention of diabetes and numerous other degenerative diseases.

---

57 Ibid.
58 Ibid.

My advice is don't worry about too many details. The important thing is to get going now. Getting the OK from your primary care physician is very important if you're just starting out.

If you are planning to use your local gym, there are a number of ways you can get cardio—the treadmill, the elliptical machine, a stair step machine, a stationary bicycle, a rowing machine, and others.

My recommendation is to start with the elliptical or stationary exercise bike as, unlike the treadmill, these do not put near as much wear and tear on the hips, knees, ankles, and lower back—not to mention tendons and ligaments.

Begin with three to five minutes and build from there until you are doing a minimum of twenty to thirty minutes or more. Learn your maximum exercise heart rate* and work to achieve about **80 percent** of that rate during your cardio workout.

2. Strength training or anaerobic exercise: the ultimate anti-aging strategy! It is true that developing and maintaining muscle mass is an important factor in longevity. Studies show that there is a co-relation between body fat composition, lean muscle mass, and longevity. Those with an ideal body fat and lean muscle mass composition enjoy much more quantity and quality of life with lower all-cause mortality.[59]

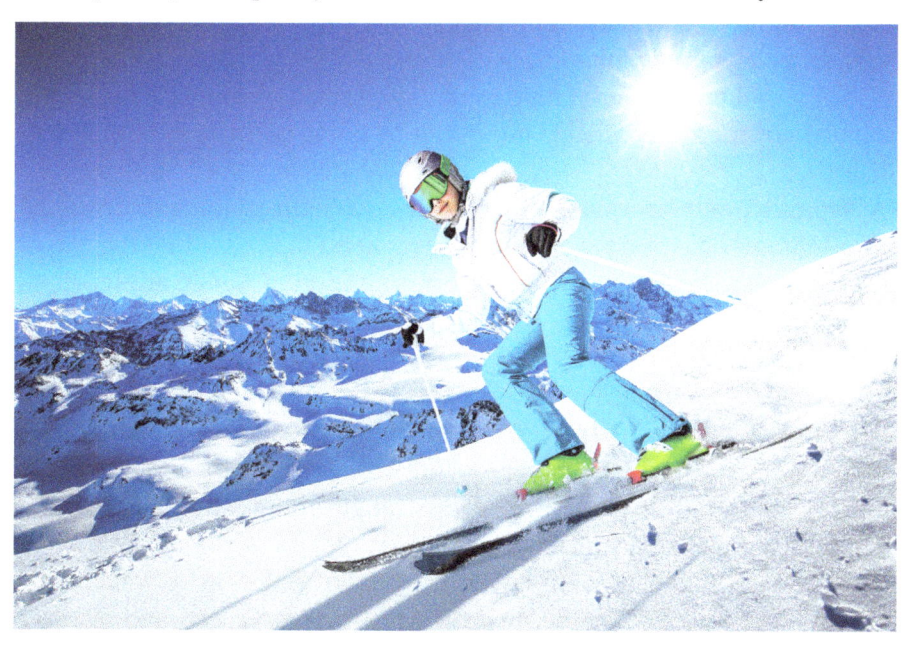

---

59 Preethi Srikanthan and Arun Karlamangla, "Muscle Mass Index as a Predictor of Longevity in Older-Adults," *The American Journal of Medicine* 127 (2014): pp. 547–553.

Individuals who work at achieving good fitness earlier in life and continue to foster it, will be rewarded in their later years in spades. They will typically be stronger and equipped to do many of the daily tasks that are required around the house as well as participate in physical activities such as walking, swimming, golf, hiking, and other indoor and outdoor pursuits. In turn, these activities will further foster good mobility and range of motion, not to mention improved circulation and cardiovascular function.

This has been my personal experience. Past my mid-sixties in age, I engage in all manner of activities including hockey, slalom skiing, golfing, hiking, and much more. Along with a plant-based diet, which I will get into in more detail in the next chapter, I am blessed with stamina and energy that often equals or exceeds those half my age! It goes without saying that being able to function well into the "golden" years gives a satisfaction and quality of life that enhances mood, happiness, fulfillment, and purpose in life.

So, if physical activity is so great, what do we mean exactly by strength training, the second important component?

Simply put, it is exercising the muscles of the body to either build or maintain healthy muscle mass.

If you are doing some sort of cardio or walking program, you are already exercising and strengthening some of the largest muscles of the body, namely your leg muscles.

These can be further built up by doing leg strengthening exercises, but we must not forget to balance things out by doing *upper body* strengthening as well.

Typically, men are more drawn to the strength training and women more so to aerobic exercise, but both sexes need to realize that the two of these, as well as flexibility training, are most important for all around good benefits and results.

A researcher, Miriam E. Nelson, PhD, created news worldwide when the results of her studies on the benefits of strength training for women were published in the Journal of the American Medical Association. Her book, *Strong Women Stay Young,* documents in detail the results of her studies. She found that after a year of strength training **twice a week for only twenty minutes**, women's bodies were *fifteen to twenty years more youthful.* Without the use of drugs, they regained bone density, which helps prevent osteoporosis. They became stronger—in most cases even stronger than when they were young. Their flexibility and balance improved. Without changing what they ate, they were leaner and trimmer. What's more, the women in her study were so energized that they became 27 percent more active.[60]

3. Flexibility training or stretching is excellent for your body. According to healthline.com, "[s]tretching your body to become more supple and flexible offers many physical benefits. Such training allows for easier and deeper movements while building strength and stability. Stretching your muscles and joints also leads to greater range of motion, improved balance, and increased flexibility.[61]

Flexibility training or stretching, like walking, is something that almost everyone can do in some way. For most people, even though they may not exercise vigorously, it is an activity that reaps many benefits. Let's look at these and other benefits in more detail.

> **1. Flexibility**—The more you stretch, the more flexible you will become. Getting up and down from the chair, getting in and out of the car, going up the stairs, reaching down to pick up something—these are all so much easier when you make it a daily habit to stretch.
>
> I often hear the excuse, "Oh, I am just getting older and with that I have become stiffer and less flexible." That is nonsense! They simply have not taken the time to stretch, and when they do, they will find that they do not have the stiffness and discomfort and can enjoy a much greater quality of life. I am living proof that stretching is a game-changer in reducing and eliminating pain, preventing injury, and improving performance in almost anything you undertake.
>
> **2. Improved Posture and Balance**—As you gain flexibility, it is quite likely your posture will improve as well. As you stretch, you work out imbalances, increase your range of motion, and achieve proper alignment.
>
> **3. Fewer Injuries**—In developing strength and flexibility, you will be able to withstand more physical stress. You will also rid your body of any muscle imbalances, which will reduce your chance of getting injured. Before a game of hockey, or any sport for that matter, I have gotten into the habit of gently stretching critical leg

---

60   Miriam Nelson, *Strong Women Stay Young* (New York, NY: Bantam Books, 1997).
61   Emily Cronkleton, "Why Being Flexible Is Great for Your Health," healthline, https://1ref.us/1qr (accessed October 28, 2021).

and groin muscles before stepping out onto the ice. Once I have warmed up, I will do an extra set of stretches before the game begins.

4. Less Pain—Many years ago, I badly injured my back by herniating the L5/S1 disc/joint in my sacroiliac spine. Add to that a mild to moderate thoracic scoliosis (curvature of the spine), osteoarthritis, and degenerative discs in the cervical spine (neck) and you have a recipe for excruciating pain. I have to thank my chiropractor and massage therapist who, at the time, gave me the proper stretches that I use to this day to keep me limber and free from most pain and stiffness. Every day, as much as I can, I will do my neck, back, and leg stretches which have made a huge difference in my overall musculoskeletal health and well-being.

5. Greater Strength and Physical Performance—Increasing strength goes hand in hand with gaining flexibility. Keeping these two areas up enables you to have the right amount of tension in the muscles so that they're strong enough to support you and your movements.

Once you increase your flexibility to allow greater movement in your body, you'll be able to perform better physically. This is what all athletes want, and you can be sure that they have a rigid stretching routine.

We have primarily dealt with physical activity, but what about mental activity? Countless studies demonstrate the close relationship between physical fitness and mental health. Physical exercise itself enhances mental function by providing greater oxygenation of the brain cells and will improve your memory, intelligence, and cognitive abilities.

Other ways to keep your "gray matter" in excellent shape are activities that include information and/or exercises to improve your performance in other meaningful endeavors. Read a book that interests or challenges you or that helps you become better or more knowledgeable in your field. Books on personal, business, and spiritual growth are excellent. Audio books and training videos also qualify. Memorization of a Bible passage or a goal, affirmation, or poem, doing jigsaw puzzles, crossword puzzles, expanding your vocabulary, or learning a new language are all examples of activities that stimulate brain function and contributes to the development of new brain cells!

Up until a few years ago, it was not believed that the brain could actually grow new brain cells to replace the ones that had died.

Now, we know from science that the brain can indeed regenerate itself and the activities listed above are just some exercises that will accomplish this. Unfortunately, watching TV typically does not stimulate new brain cells or exercise the brain so be careful to limit your TV or computer time.[62]

Remember, if we don't exercise our brain cells on a *daily* basis, they die. An extensive study involved more than 2,800 participants over the age of sixty-five who each engaged in one of three different forms of cognitive training. Types of training used included speed of processing training, memory training, and reasoning training. The results showed the speed-of-processing group experienced the greatest benefits, but all three groups benefitted, experiencing protection from age-related cognitive declines that lasted at least five years.[63] It goes to show that brain health is no exception when it comes to the old saying, "If you don't use it, you'll lose it."

Extra TRANSFORMational Tips for Activity:

It may be a relief for you to know that scientific evidence clearly shows that moderate-intensity activity is all that is required to enjoy the greatest benefits of exercise. We don't have to be marathon runners or pump iron for hours to receive all the health benefits named above. Any regular exercise/activity will be beneficial.

Are time constraints making it difficult to get your workout in?

Consider **high-intensity interval training or HIIT**. There are numerous routines along these lines, but the general principle is alternating short periods of

It may be a relief for you to know that scientific evidence clearly shows that moderate-intensity activity is all that is required to enjoy the greatest benefits of exercise. We don't have to be marathon runners or pump iron for hours to receive all the health benefits named above.

---

62 Brian Mastroianni, "Binge-Watching TV May Be Dulling Your Brain," healthline, https://1ref.us/1qs (accessed October 28, 2021).
63 Walter R. Boot and Arthur F. Kramer, "The Brain-Games Conundrum: Does Cognitive Training Really Sharpen the Mind?" NCBI, https://1ref.us/1qt (accessed October 28, 2021).

intense anaerobic or strength exercise followed by less vigorous recovery periods.

Typically, these sessions vary from four to thirty minutes (e.g., eight cycles of twenty seconds of intense anaerobic and ten seconds of less intense aerobic exercise). These short, powerful workouts provide improved athletic conditioning, glucose metabolism, and fat burning.

In testing, it was generally determined that this strategy, while taking much less time, gave as good, if not better, overall results than continuous training over a longer period of time.

Exercising properly can help men and women build natural testosterone in the body.

In my practice, I treat a lot of patients struggling with hormonal imbalances. Oftentimes, I work with men to help them to naturally build testosterone, which is vital for sex drive or libido, preventing erectile dysfunction (ED), improving mood, muscle strength, and motivation.

The mistake that many men over forty make is that they will do thirty minutes or so of cardio and then hit the weights. Unfortunately, anything over five minutes or so of cardio will somewhat reduce or shut off testosterone production completely. When weightlifting follows the cardio, during which the bulk of testosterone is normally produced, it is of little benefit.

The solution is to do your weights one day and cardio the next. You get good, natural testosterone production on your anaerobic, strength training day and it provides you a day in between the weights for you to recover. On that recovery day, you can do all the aerobic or cardio exercise you like.

The Mini Trampoline

Patients will ask me what I feel is the best overall exercise and I will tell them walking, as mentioned above. But for a relatively small investment, a mini trampoline is hard to beat and will pay back huge dividends.

Using a mini trampoline or rebounder is something pretty much anyone can do. It is excellent cardio, and is one of the most beneficial exercises for improving lymphatic drainage and circulation. It strengthens, conditions, and tones the legs, thighs, buttocks, and abs.

A new study, published in the International Journal of Sports Science, has concluded that rebounding exercise is twice as effective at improving aerobic fitness and 50 percent more efficient at burning fat than running.[64]

Besides giving you quick results, rebounding is fun! Make sure you get a good quality unit with good spring to it. Start out slow—maybe just a few minutes. Work up to fifteen to twenty minutes daily doing three to five-minute sessions at different times throughout the day. If you go too long in the beginning, you can feel quite fatigued, weak, and dizzy. This is just an indication of how good this method of exercise is to stimulate cleansing in the body and to help toxin elimination. You also find out very quickly whether or not you are in good physical shape. Happy bouncing!

To calculate your maximum exercise heart rate, subtract your age from 220. For example, if you are forty-five years old, subtract forty-five from 220 to get a maximum heart rate of 175. This is the average maximum number of times your heart should beat per minute during exercise.

Always consult your healthcare practitioner for advice as to whether any exercise plans would be appropriate for you or not.

---

[64] *International Journal of Sport Science*, "New Study: Rebounding Burns Fat And Improves Cardio Better Than Running," bellicon, https://1ref.us/1qu (accessed October 28, 2021).

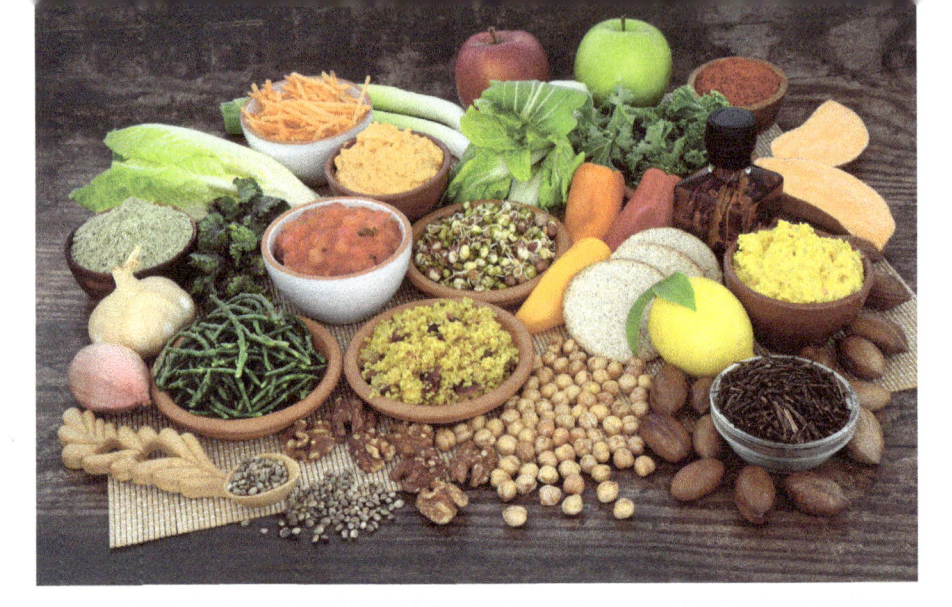

N is for ... Nutrition

Nutrition is close to the middle of TRANSFORM and for good reason. What we eat has a more profound impact on our life and health than most realize. But the problem is that when you ask anyone from a nutritional expert to your average armchair nutritionist, you are going to get a different answer each time! How confusing is that?!

Many years ago, I was directed by the hand of God to make somewhat drastic changes to my diet and lifestyle, which have held me in good stead for over forty years now. Here is the clear counsel from the Word of God (the Bible) itself. As God placed Adam and Eve in the Garden of Eden, He said, "See, I have given you every herb *that* yields seed which *is* on the face of all the earth, and every tree whose fruit yields seed; to you it shall be for food" (Gen. 1:29).

From this Scripture in the Bible, it is clear that it was God's plan for us from the beginning to eat a natural, healthy whole-food, plant-based diet that would provide for us all the elements required for a healthy, strong body, mind, and spirit ... yes, spirit, because the closer we come to the Edenic diet, not only do we experience better physical, mental, and emotional health but *spiritual health and growth* as well.

It is not my wish to go into *all* the scientific evidence here that conclusively proves that, from a health standpoint, a plant-based diet is a significantly better choice than a meat-based diet. One of the most influential documentaries of our time that has changed people's minds about whether or not to adopt a plant-based diet is *The Game Changers*,[65] which can be seen on different streaming platforms. James Wilks travels the world on a quest for the truth about meat, protein, and strength. It features elite athletes, special ops soldiers, and visionary scientists. The purpose of the documentary is to change the way people eat and live.

Suffice to say, compared to a meat-based diet, if you eat a healthy, whole-food, plant-based diet, you can expect to live longer. A study begun in 1958 and still not completed is being done on Seventh-day Adventists, many of whom have adopted a plant-based diet of varying degrees. All in all, results so far suggest, on average, vegetarian men live nine-and-a-half years longer and women a little over six years.[66] Not only do those eating a plant-based diet live longer but they also enjoy more quality of life, having a significant reduction and prevention in major degenerative diseases such as cancer, cardiovascular disease, and diabetes—and experience more stamina and athletic performance into their sixties and beyond.[67] In short, they grow old with fewer health issues.

So, let's unpack this a bit more and analyze what a good plant-based diet looks like. First of all, there are some fundamentals to cover. There is more to it than "we are what we eat." We are ultimately what we digest, assimilate, metabolize, and eliminate.

For some people, they eat, digest, assimilate, metabolize, and eliminate their food just fine, but for many others, this process does not run like a perfectly tuned race car engine or a beautiful symphony orchestra. In fact, if just *one* of these areas is "out of tune," to reference the symphony idea, the rest of our digestive system gets soured and we do not make beautiful music. Your digestion will just not function very smoothly at all.

For many, years of atrocious, abusive eating habits have undermined and degenerated the whole digestive process. Past the actual eating of the food, the mechanism of digestion has been disturbed and the person experiences a painful, laborious, tortuous, and torturous movement of food through the gastrointestinal (GI) tract.

Along the way, due to poor breakdown of the food elements, the damaged intestinal lining, and the unbalanced microbiota in the gut, all sorts of gastrointestinal disasters are created. These can include gas, bloating,

---

65   James Wilks, *The Game Changers*, Directed by Louie Psihoyos: September 16, 2019 (Germany), https://1ref.us/1qv (accessed October 28, 2021).

66   Annie Hauser, "Vegetarians Live Longer, Study Finds," *Wellness*, https://1ref.us/1qw (accessed October 28, 2021).

67   Carra Richling, "Plant-Based Eating: Getting the Right Nutrition," ornish lifestyle medicine, https://1ref.us/1qx (accessed October 28, 2021).

diarrhea, irritable bowel syndrome, food sensitivity, Crohn's disease, colitis, pancreatitis, constipation, "leaky gut syndrome," small intestinal bacteria overgrowth (SIBO), gastroesophageal reflux disease (GERD), yeast overgrowth (primarily Candida albicans) and yes, chronic parasitosis.

It is no wonder that according to a survey done in 2013, 72 percent of Americans are living with digestive symptoms like diarrhea, gas, bloating, and abdominal pain.[68]

Overall annual healthcare expenditures for gastrointestinal disease in the USA totals $136 billion, which is more than for heart disease ($113 billion), trauma ($103 billion), or mental health ($99 billion). Three million hospital admissions for GI diseases occur annually.[69]

In practice, I see these situations almost every day and an individual with these challenges needs help to sort out these issues before they can get to first base nutritionally. It is important to remember that without a good digestive process, a person cannot enjoy good health. We will discuss more on how to correct and prevent digestive challenges later in the chapter as well as in the next letter—S.

It's hard to know where to begin when detailing the widely researched benefits of a well-balanced and varied plant-based diet. As we have referred to above, scores of scientific research show marked reductions in obesity, heart disease, cancer, diabetes, and a host of other degenerative conditions. For example, Dr. Hans Diehl, founder of the Coronary Health Improvement Project (CHIP), compares the foods with the worst health outcomes—such as meats, dairy, eggs, processed foods, alcohol, and caffeine which lead to disease progression—to the foods with the best health outcomes. These are fruits and vegetables, whole grains, legumes, some nuts and seeds, and water. These foods lead to disease reversal.[70]

So ... assuming we are digesting, assimilating, metabolizing, and eliminating our food well, what should and should we not eat?

What we should eat is simple. As Genesis 1:29 indicates, eat largely of fresh fruits, vegetables, nuts, seeds, legumes, and whole grains grown as naturally as possible and most preferably in the locale in which you live. Avoid, wherever possible, genetically modified (GMO) foods, commercially grown, pesticide- and herbicide-laden foods.

---

68 "New Survey Reveals More than Half of Americans are Living with Gastrointestinal Symptoms and Not Seeking Care from a Doctor," abbvie, https://1ref.us/1qy (accessed October 28, 2021).
69 John R. Saltzman, reviewing Peery AF et al., "Burden and cost of gastrointestinal, liver and pancreatic diseases in the United States," *Gastroenterology*, https://1ref.us/1qz (accessed October 28, 2021).
70 Chef AJ, "Can Heart Disease be Reversed? | Interview with Dr. Hans Diehl," https://1ref.us/1r0 (accessed October 28, 2021).

Organically grown foods are most preferred and are becoming more and more available. Prices are gradually coming down closer to regular produce prices. In an *Associated Press* article in January of 2019, it stated, "Last year, organic food and beverages cost an average of 24 cents more per unit than conventional food, or about 7.5 percent more, according to Nielsen. That was down from a 27 cent, or 9 percent, premium in 2014."[71] Now, there is a lot of variation within these figures, but overall, as more supply comes to market, the prices will continue to fall.

The main benefits for choosing organically grown foods are the following:

1. **Organic foods are free of harmful pesticides, antibiotics, GMOs, and food additives like preservatives, colorings, flavorings, MSG, and artificial sweeteners**. Organically grown foods must comply with strict standards to assure customers that they are indeed organically grown. There is much research data on why we want to avoid these chemicals, but in short, there is growing evidence that concentrated pesticide exposures, for example, are related to increased rates of chronic diseases like diabetes and cancer—particularly lymphoma and Alzheimer's. Women are especially at risk as there are links to breast cancer due to pesticides mimicking estrogen in the body—a known breast cancer risk factor. Furthermore, exposure to certain types of pesticides can decrease fertility, pose risk for sperm abnormalities, cause a decrease in male births, initiate spontaneous abortion and birth defects or fetal growth retardation.[72] Men also are more susceptible to prostate cancer with the intake of pesticide-laden food and the absorption of these estrogen-like compounds.

2. **They have less of an environmental impact than conventional farming**. Many years of synthetic chemical commercial fertilizers, which are bereft of all but three minerals, have, unfortunately, depleted and eroded soils significantly. It is estimated that today, roughly 100 trace minerals and elements are deficient in human diets in most regions of the world.[73]

   If we could but fathom how the deficiency of just one of these trace elements creates numerous health conditions, imagine how

---

71 "Good news if you buy organic food—it's getting cheaper," Associated Press, January 24, 2019.
72 Linda M. Frazier, "Reproductive disorders associated with pesticide exposure," J Agromedicine 12 (2007), https://1ref.us/1r1 (accessed October 28, 2021).
73 Ward Chesworth, Felipe Macias-Vasquez, David Acquaye and Edmond Thompson, "Agriculture Alchemy: Stones into Bread," Episodes - *Journal of International Geoscience* 1983, p. 5.

the deficiency of 100 trace minerals would affect human health. The widespread and serious problem of soil erosion and de-mineralization has been vastly exacerbated in this century by governmental policies that support widespread deforestation, massive monoculture cropping, and heavy agrochemical dependency.[74]

According to the United Nations, the groundwater in many agricultural areas is polluted with synthetic fertilizers and pesticides.[75] Organic farming greatly reduces the threat of water pollution and prevents damage due to soil erosion while at the same time, if done correctly, re-mineralizing the soil.

3. **Higher nutritional value.** A number of studies have been done over the years regarding this particular issue. Some studies completed eight or more years ago claimed there was no difference between foods commercially grown with pesticides, herbicides, and synthetic fertilizer and those grown organically. Today, the evidence is overwhelming in favor of organic food. The results from an analysis of 343 peer-reviewed studies from around the world—more than ever before—was done and published in a respected scientific journal, the *British Journal of Nutrition*.[76] The study examined the differences between organic and conventional fruit, vegetables, and cereals. "The crucially important thing about this research is that it shatters the myth that how we farm does not affect the quality of the food we eat," said Helen Browning, chief executive of Soil Association. The analysis found that organic food has more antioxidant compounds ranging from 19 to 69 percent higher than non-organic foods, which are associated with "a reduced risk of chronic diseases, including cardiovascular diseases, neurodegenerative diseases and certain cancers."[77] As stated above, with proper organic growing methods, the foods will contain a better trace mineral composition which is vital to our health as well.

---

74 Raymond Obomsawin, "Pathogenic Microbes and Disease: Causation or Consequences?" April 2020, p. 13.
75 "Agriculture: cause and victim of water pollution, but change is possible," Food and Agriculture Organization of the United Nations, https://1ref.us/1r2 (accessed October 28, 2021).
76 Monte Morin, "Organic foods are more nutritious according to review of 343 studies," *Los Angeles Times*, https://1ref.us/1r3 (accessed October 28, 2021).
77 Damian Carrington and George Arnett, "Clear Differences between organic and non-organic food, study finds," *The Guardian*, https://1ref.us/1r4 (accessed October 28, 2021).

4. **Safer meat**. For those who choose to eat meat, organic meat is raised without antibiotics, hormones, or food treated with pesticides.[78]

5. **More economical**. When you consider eating organically, you are likely more mindful of what you are putting into your mouth and the mouths of your family. This often translates into a shifting of your food choices and, ultimately, your grocery bill. What I am getting at here is instead of eating out or ordering fast food, you are more likely to favor your own organic food. You will create a cost difference that will, in all probability, end up costing you less.

What we should avoid are foods that were once considered a very occasional treat but have now crept into our diet and become staple foods. Examples are sugar (the current average amount of sugar Americans eat daily in teaspoons in their food is 42.5!),[79] including cakes, pies, cookies, muffins, candy bars (and other bars that are loaded with sugar), ice cream, milk chocolate, soft drinks, refined white flour and breads, cereal, pastas, fried foods, caffeinated beverages and foods, high-fat foods, hydrogenated and partially hydrogenated oils and foods containing them.

A plant-based, anti-inflammatory diet avoids or strictly limits dairy products, commercially grown wheat, soy, corn, and citrus since these are commonly at the root of many people's intestinal complaints due to sensitivity, inflammation, lactose intolerance, and so on.

Most snacks and junk food contained in "crinkly" packages are often loaded with high-calorie hydrogenated fat, salt, sugar, commercially grown potatoes, white flour, and GMO corn.

Families are so busy these days; they are going out to eat more than ever before. They often choose fast-food restaurants, which, by and large, can be nutritional nightmares if you are not **very** careful!

Is it any wonder we are teetering on the edge of ruin as our country plunges into chronic degenerative diseases such as obesity, diabetes, cancer, and cardiovascular disease like never before? As of the writing of this book, the world has been thrust into a very controversial COVID-19 pandemic. With the above conditions as a backdrop, seasonal flu or viruses are deadly to people suffering with these ailments. With these comorbidities compromising their immune systems, they succumb because their

---

[78] "Pros and cons of organic foods," Jen's Modest Treasures, https://1ref.us/1r5 (accessed October 28, 2021).

[79] "How Much Sugar Do You Eat? You May Be Surprised!" https://1ref.us/1r6 (accessed October 28, 2021).

weakened, dysfunctional immune system overreacts and wreaks havoc on their system. The overreaction of a dysfunctional immune system is what ultimately is responsible for their demise, not the virus.

In fact, as a result of poor diet, coupled with lack of activity leading to obesity and obesity-related diseases, we are told that too many of the current generation may, on average, live less healthy and possibly even shorter lives than their parents.[80]

Obesity itself has eclipsed all other diseases and conditions by becoming the number one health problem that we Canadians and Americans face. And contrary to popular belief, **diet**—not exercise—is the best method to release weight. I tell my patients the secret to reducing weight is achieved by 80 percent diet and 20 percent exercise. It is also important to remember that you cannot "out-exercise a bad diet!"

One of the foundational specialties that we have provided in our clinics is weight loss or weight release. For years, I pondered how it was that people gained weight. There seemed to be no good explanation anywhere, especially when some people didn't seem to eat any more than before, exercised regularly, and either couldn't lose an ounce or stubbornly still gained weight.

Many years ago, I had adopted the Atkins diet in my clinic, and although I abandoned it because of its obvious flaws, it really did work. That set me to thinking about why it worked so well. It wasn't until some years later that I came to the real reason people gained weight. What I am going to share with you now is the underlying cause of our number one health problem in North America.

Weight gain is primarily a **hormonal** problem. By far, the hormone most responsible is insulin, followed to a somewhat lesser degree by cortisol. For most people, when I tell them this fact, I get a blank look like I was speaking to them in a different language. What do hormones have to do with gaining weight? Well, as it turns out, it has everything to do with it.

Here's how the majority of us gain weight. In North America today, we love to eat way too many carbohydrates. Carbohydrate foods are found in abundance in our diet. They are often consumed because they are "comfort" foods that appeal to our tastebuds, our "sweet-tooth," and are relatively inexpensive. Carbohydrates, or "carbs," are divided into two main groups—simple and complex carbs. Simple carbs are found in fruits, fruit juices, soft drinks, alcohol, honey, maple syrup, high fructose corn

---

80 S. Jay Olshansky et al., "A Potential Decline in Life Expectancy in the United States in the 21st Century," *The New England Journal of Medicine* 352 (2005), https://1ref.us/1r7 (accessed October 28, 2021).

syrup, and sugar. They can also be found in all foods containing sugar like sweets, desserts, cookies, ice cream, chocolate bars, and many other sugary foods. Complex carbs are found in starchy root vegetables like potatoes, sweet potatoes, beets, carrots, and others. They are also found in nuts, seeds, and legumes, which consist of chickpeas, soybeans and other beans, split peas, lentils, carob, peanuts, and tamarind. Other complex carbs are found in grains such as wheat, oats, and barley, as well as corn.

When we consume any type of carbohydrate, the body converts it to a simple sugar called glucose. In order to metabolize that sugar, or glucose, into the cells, the pancreas produces **insulin.** The amount of insulin produced depends on the amount of carbs consumed and the resulting glucose that needs to be metabolized.

Because, as a population, we are consuming so many carbohydrates, the pancreas is producing much more insulin than in times past. Normally, the pancreas meters out insulin in small amounts as needed, but with so many carbs being consumed daily, the pancreas has to abandon the slow and measured amounts of insulin and it pours out the insulin like there's no tomorrow.

It would be interesting to compare from 1900 till now how much sugar consumption has risen. Estimates vary, but as far as we can tell, in 1900 the average person consumed about 90 lbs. per year and in 2009 that figure had risen to nearly 180 lbs. per year.[81] This number is rising every year so twelve years later, as of the writing of this book, we are sure to be five to ten or more pounds higher than that. Now, our pancreas has to produce double or more the amount of insulin than the early 1900s.

This extra wear and tear on the pancreas and the exorbitant amounts of sugar trying to enter the cells eventually causes insulin resistance, hyperglycemia, and a relative lack of insulin which has led to an unprecedented level of type 2 diabetes (T2D). Many people who are overweight are at a greater risk of developing this crippling disease. A lot of them are moving toward prediabetes.

With all these carbs in the blood, we create what is called hyperinsulinemia, which is simply excess insulin pouring out of the pancreas to metabolize all the sugar (carbs). Because the insulin is not metered out to meet the demand, there will always be excess insulin left over once all the sugar/glucose has been delivered to the cells.

It is this *excess* insulin that now becomes the problem with weight gain. Simply stated, this leftover insulin (hyperinsulinemia) will cause damage

---

[81] Kamila Laura Sitwell, "Sugar consumption now vs 100 years ago," LinkedIn, https://1ref.us/1r8 (accessed October 28, 2021).

to the tissue and so the body creates extra fat cells to engulf the insulin to protect the body from damage. In this way, as each day, week, and month passes, you are continually adding more fat so that eventually you see your weight creeping up and up over time.

The answer to reverse this situation and release the fat and insulin that has been engulfed is to lower carbs, lower fats, and make sure protein levels are adequate. By doing this, your body is able to go into ketosis or "fat-burning" mode. Our body's default form of energy is carbohydrates, which we normally get from our diet. This energy, among other things, is used to maintain body heat, to provide for the proper functioning of the brain, and to fuel the muscles. When we reduce carbs, the body will draw upon stored glucose or glycogen mainly found in the muscles. Once that is gone, the body will search for another source of energy for fuel.

It is of paramount importance at this time that we provide enough protein to spare lean muscle, or the body will pull protein out of the muscle to provide energy for survival. Once this is looked after, the body will seek out the only other meaningful source of energy left, which is your body fat. After about three to four days of this strategy, your body will make the switch to ketosis and tap into your body fat for its main source of energy.

Contrary to what some might say, ketosis has been widely researched and found to be beneficial and safe, even for extended periods of time.[82]

Think about it. Once a person is in full ketosis, it is truly a wonderful thing. While in fat-burning mode, your body is burning your own body fat twenty-four hours a day, seven days a week! For most people, their energy increases because fat delivers almost double the energy per gram consumed.

The health benefits are enormous. We see almost universal resolution of gastric reflux, stomach and intestinal gas, and other GI symptoms, insomnia, reduced or normalized blood pressure, joint pain, normalized blood sugar levels, normalized blood cholesterol and lipid levels. Cravings disappear or are greatly reduced, and you experience a feeling of satiation.

By following this plan, you are greatly decreasing the requirement for insulin and thereby resting the pancreas, releasing excess fat and sparing your lean muscle mass. This is indeed the proper way to release weight. Why? Because the weight you want to release is not muscle but the excess fat that you have accumulated.

---

[82] Hussein M. Dashti et al., "Long-term effects of a ketogenic diet in obese patients," *Experimental and Clinical Cardiology* 9 (2004): pp. 200-205.

Sad but true, most diets from the worst to the more respected ones actually create a situation where you can lose as much lean muscle mass as you do fat. Losing lean muscle is not desirable for a number of reasons:

1. Your lean muscle is the *furnace* that burns calories in your body. The leaner the muscle mass, the more calories you burn; the less muscle mass you have, the less you burn.

2. Your lean muscle mass not only helps to prevent obesity but is directly co-related to your longevity. The leaner your muscle mass, the more likely you are to live a longer and more quality life.

3. After the age of thirty, our muscle mass begins to degenerate. On average, between the ages of forty to sixty, a person gains about one pound of fat and loses a half pound of muscle per year. By the age of seventy-five, up to 50 percent of our muscle mass can vanish.[83] Gradually, we lose strength and mobility. Thankfully, God made us so that we can rebuild muscle mass through diet and exercise if we are intentional about it.

4. Greater muscle mass reduces the risk of falls and injuries. The greater the amount of muscle mass, the higher bone mineral density you will have. Dense, strong bones prevent injuries and fractures, but lean muscle mass does more than just strengthen our bones, it also stabilizes and strengthens our joints.

5. Greater muscle mass gives an improved quality of life. Building lean muscle improves many aspects of our physical

> *Building lean muscle improves many aspects of our physical health, but it also positively influences our emotional and mental health. Those who consistently invest in their lean muscle mass enjoy better sleep, more energy, and greater self-esteem, as well as less stress and depression.*

---

83 Mark H. Beers and Robert Berkow, *The Merck Manual of Geriatrics* (Whitehouse Station, NJ: Merck Research Laboratories, 2009), See esp. chapters 31, 48, and 66.

health, but it also positively influences our emotional and mental health. Those who consistently invest in their lean muscle mass enjoy better sleep, more energy, and greater self-esteem, as well as less stress and depression.[84]

Later on in this chapter, I will provide you with a simple weight reduction plan.

How to Improve Digestion

Some principles to follow to enable optimum digestion are the following:

- Always eat in a relaxed, unhurried, pleasant atmosphere.
- Pause before eating to return thanks to God.
- Chew your food slowly and thoroughly and avoid washing it down with fluids.
- Eat until 80 percent full rule—known as "systematic under eating."
- If you are not hungry, wait until you are. If you are hungry before bed, best to have a large glass of water or piece of fruit and wake up to enjoy a sumptuous breakfast.
- Avoid combining fruits and vegetables, carbs and fats.
- Avoid snacks if possible and allow four to five hours between meals.
- Use the "pushback" rule—stop eating, push back from the table, and start clearing dishes. For the men—your wife will love it and so will the weigh scale.
- Light activity is best after a meal—lying down after is decidedly harmful.
- Drink unlimited water between meals and very little with meals.
- Use bitter herbs or specific strain probiotics to help digestion and reduce intestinal gas.

Improving digestion varies from individual to individual. It can take some years to correct it and feel better.

---

[84] News Company, "5 Benefits of Lean Muscle Mass Besides a Good Physique," https://1ref.us/1r9 (accessed October 28, 2021).

Extra TRANSFORMational Tips for Nutrition:

Simple Weight Reduction Plan:

At the outset, men will typically release weight easier than women.

For breakfast, I recommend a meal replacement, plant-based protein shake with no more than twelve to eighteen grams carbohydrates and reasonably low fat. For lunch and dinner, follow the plant-based, anti-inflammatory diet (mentioned earlier in this chapter in the section on organically grown food being more economical) with an emphasis on four cups maximum (two cups at each meal or four cups at either meal) of low glycemic* vegetables, unlimited lettuce and other greens, and four to six ounces of plant-based protein entrees.

Allow no more than four hours between meals. For example, if you have breakfast at 8 a.m., you should be eating by noon or earlier. If you eat lunch at noon and have supper at 6 p.m., you have a gap of six hours which is somewhat more than the four-hour rule. To prevent low blood sugar and its potential to cause cravings and other undesirable symptoms, have a snack at three or so in the afternoon to break up that long six-hour period. The snack can be some raw, low-glycemic veggies, or low-carb, plant-based protein. *No fruit* allowed in the weight release phase.

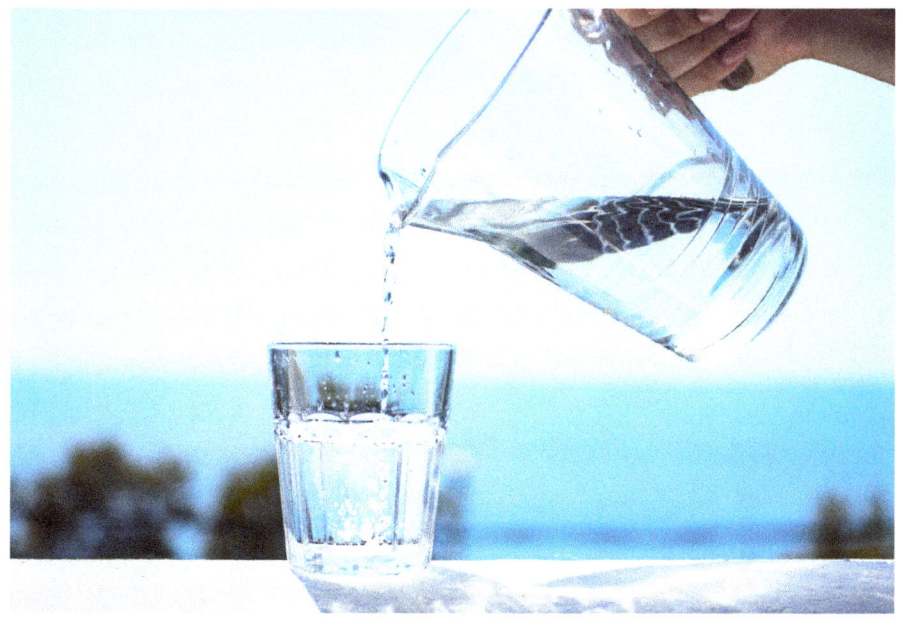

Water is another important secret weapon in successfully reducing weight.

Drink a *minimum* of eight glasses of water daily, drink one to two cups of an herbal slimming, cleansing tea (without caffeine), and watch the weight melt off. Do *light to moderate* walking, cycling, etc. three to five days a week for twenty to thirty minutes maximum.

For women, have the same low-carb, plant-based protein shake for breakfast recommended for men above. For lunch and dinner, reduce carbs and fats, eat four cups daily of low glycemic veggies plus unlimited lettuce and greens, avoid grains, starchy foods, fruits, fruit juices, and eat good low-carb, plant-based protein foods as mentioned above.

Follow the four-hour rule as mentioned above as well as snack suggestions except for fruit. Drink a *minimum* eight glasses water daily and no exercise other than your usual daily activities until you have reached your goal weight. You will love the new, healthy, and vibrant you!

*The glycemic index is a figure representing the relative ability of a carbohydrate food to increase the level of glucose in the blood. Pretty much all foods have been given a number. The higher the number, the more that food will increase glucose in the blood. While you are releasing weight, you want to choose foods that are low on the glycemic index (GI). The GI can be found by clicking on the URL to our website below: https://www.sloannaturalhealthcenter.com

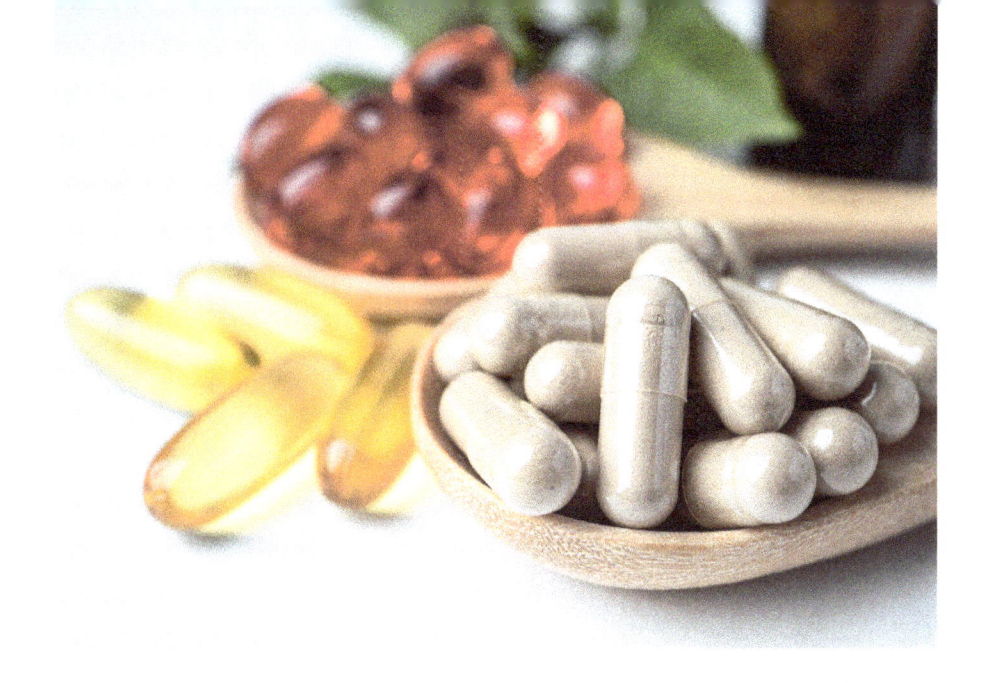

S is for ... Supplementation

In all my years of practice, it has been very clear to me that **supplementation** (the use of concentrated superfoods, vitamins, minerals, herbs, homeopathic remedies, nutritional, herbal and homeopathic complexes and formulas) of natural products to the diet can make a huge difference in quality of life, disease prevention, anti-aging, and life extension.

My healthiest patients over the years are generally those who wisely and generously have used supplements in addition to a healthy diet and lifestyle.

Many years ago, the point was driven home to me by a patient upon whom I made house calls. This woman was 103 years old and did not take *any* over-the-counter drugs or prescriptions! I soon discovered that she shunned these things and instead had a battery of herbal and vitamin supplements that she used regularly. In fact, her daughter, who was in her early eighties, who I also looked after, was not nearly as healthy or as spry as her mom, nor was she as diligent or focused on natural ways of health.

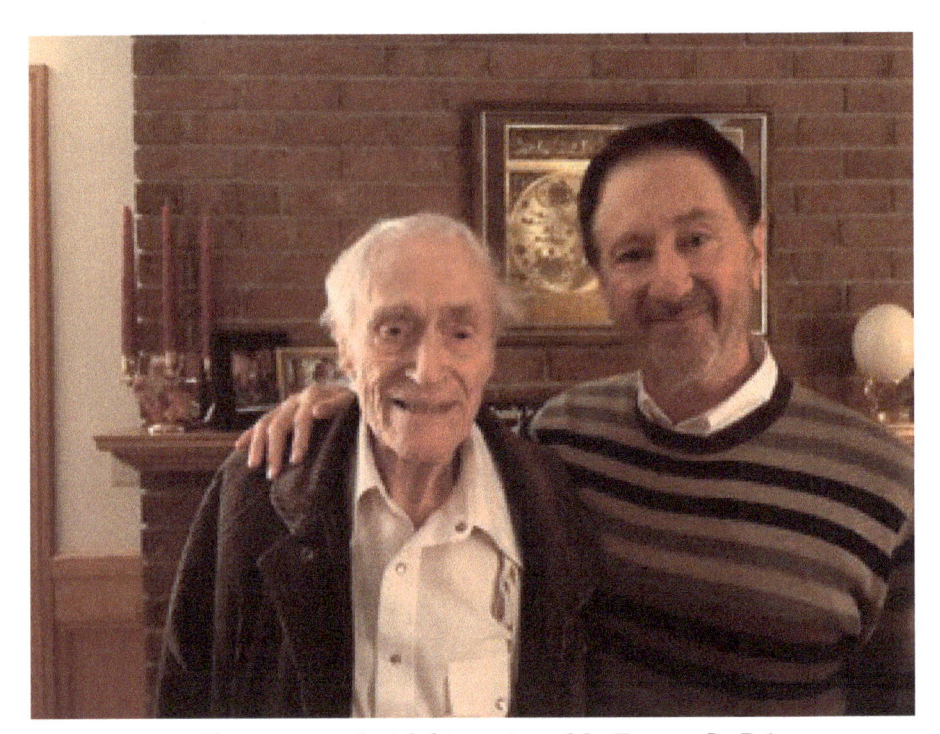

Dr. Sloan pictured with his patient, Mr. Eugene LaBrie, on the occasion of his 100th birthday in March of 2020

    This made a lasting impression on me and has been reinforced many times over through the years. My oldest current patient, who just turned 100 years old, came to me in his late eighties and gave me the mandate that I was to help him live as long as possible. At the time, he was full of vim and vigor and could outwork most people half his age. He, too, did not take any prescriptions or over-the-counter medications but, instead, chose to utilize nutrition, hard work, and natural remedies for any of his ills. It is wonderful to see that, more than a decade later, his family physician, upon reviewing his latest battery of blood tests, called him a physical superstar!

    For those of you who may think, "Well, he is just one of those with an abnormally outstanding constitution," it is important to note that my patient took pains to explain to me that he had been plagued with numerous health crises throughout his life but was able to work his way through them by adopting careful dietary and lifestyle practices. Indeed, over this time I have had the privilege to look after him, we have dealt with numerous health challenges, all by applying natural health practices, supplements, and treatments.

The Case for Supplementation

The monumental depletion of nutrients in the soil over the decades due to agribusiness and aggressive, non-sustainable farming methods has left the nutritional value of our soil and foods drastically depleted compared to a mere twenty or thirty years ago.

Add to that the tens of thousands of toxic synthetic chemicals and heavy metals released into our environment every day and the tons and tons of pesticides and herbicides sprayed on our food. We need to include the fast-increasing exposure to radiation from electromagnetic frequencies (EMF), e.g., new generations of cellular networks that are largely untested for their potential damaging impact on the human system, smartphones, computer screens, Wi-Fi, and microwave towers.

Last but not least, we can't forget the ravages of stressful and sedentary lifestyles on our health as well. All of the above serves to give us the perfect storm for serious illness—cancer, heart disease, and arthritis as well as the rise in autoimmune disorders such as multiple sclerosis (MS), Hashimoto's thyroiditis, psoriasis, inflammatory bowel disease (IBD), rheumatoid arthritis, and others.

Respiratory disorders, hormone disruption and imbalance, and Lyme disease are also very possible because of living in a very toxic world. I might add that these issues are *not* just the result of living longer or due to old age. All of these are seen across the entire age spectrum, and most unfortunately, even in our young children.

Furthermore, our fruits and vegetables are often harvested before they are ripe, gassed with ethylene, gathered in distribution warehouses, prepared, and shipped by truck all over the continent and, in some cases, globally. When it arrives, it is unloaded into another distribution center and then shipped to the various grocery outlets in that region. Fruits like apples and pears and most root vegetables can be kept for months in cold storage but this has been found to reduce the cancer-preventative benefits and antioxidant activity of fruits and vegetables. An important measure you can take to reduce the impact of the sprays is to use a fruit and vegetable detergent spray to wash the surface of the fruit or vegetable, even if they are organic.

Once it gets to the grocery store, it is then unpacked and placed out in the light and air in the produce department. By the time the consumer gets it, it could have been up to a week or more since it was harvested, thereby continuing to lose additional nutritional value during this time.

Now, we take that produce home and what do we do with it? Well, we put it in the fridge and eat it here and there over the week. Often, we deplete our food even more by improper and overcooking methods.

By the time your food makes it into your stomach, the overall nutritional value would have been diminished considerably compared to if it was harvested fresh out of your own garden and eaten right then.

What we have created is a paradox—even though we have more than enough to eat, many of us are actually malnourished. Without adequate vitamins, minerals, enzymes, essential fatty acids, and amino acids, the body begins to struggle to keep in balance and we begin to see physical, mental, and emotional symptoms present themselves.

Add the ever-constant stress to the mix and these symptoms can intensify. Our body systems start to break down. We don't feel well. We find ourselves getting sick more often; our digestion becomes troublesome; we lose energy and find ourselves tired more and more of the time.

Despite the fact that the Lord has created us to be marvelously equipped with many systems to eliminate wastes, impurities, toxins etc., over time, exposure to *all* of these abovementioned assaults begins to take its toll on the eliminatory capacity of the body, and symptoms of toxicity can emerge.

First, there can be vague symptoms of feeling run-down, fatigued, sluggish, irritated, gas, bloating, less resistance to illness, skin problems, etc., which can accumulate and become more and more of a problem as time goes on.

Oftentimes, a cold or fever with flu symptoms is simply your body taking action and burning off accumulated impurities in your system. I have often told my patients with colds over the years that they were experiencing a good "cleanse." In fact, when someone comes down with a cold or a flu virus, it's not the virus that's at fault, it is actually caused by a dysfunctional immune system. There are countless viruses around us all the time; so, if the virus was at fault, we would be sick *all the time*.

When we do succumb, it is because we are **immunocompromised** which can be a result of old age, pre-existing health conditions or comorbidities, poor diet, lifestyle, lack of sleep, stress, and so on. When exposed to a virus, the weakened immune system *overreacts* and this overreaction is what causes the damage, leading to more severe symptoms and in some cases even death.

If you are experiencing some of what we have been describing in the last few pages and a checkup with your doctor shows very little, if anything wrong, what you *really* need is a tune-up or a body cleanse.

Just like you wash and cleanse the outside of your body, it shouldn't seem particularly unusual to cleanse the inside as well. In order to do this correctly, I recommend it be done in a systematic way—**daily cleansing** and **periodic cleansing.** Daily cleansing can be achieved with an herbal blend[85] that gently cleanses the whole body.

Periodic cleansing can take many forms, but the idea is to focus on an area of the body to flush out. Typically the focus is on an organ of elimination like the bowel or the kidneys that can get congested over time and thus increase the risk of disease. Because my complete recovery depended on detoxing my own body, detoxification or body cleansing has been a hallmark of my practice from the earliest days. It has proven over and over to significantly improve health status. If you want to achieve optimal health, it is a must.

Every day, if possible, I recommend taking the following supplements to support the body nutritionally, immunologically, and ecologically:

- Herbal body-cleansing tea
- Multiple vitamin and mineral
- Antioxidant formula
- Probiotic for maintaining healthy intestinal flora
- Trace mineral drops added to purified water
- Omega-3 essential fatty acids from ground flax, hemp, or chia (oils expressed from these in capsule form is best)
- Concentrated greens formula
- Male or female support formula for hormone balance and reproductive gland health (breast, ovaries, uterus in women; prostate and testes in men). Begin around age thirty
- Immune boosting formula
- Fiber supplement
- Iodine or kelp
- Vitamin D3—minimum 2,000 to 5,000 IUs daily. The darker your skin, the more you will need. RDAs for vitamin D is restricted to 1,000 IUs per day but this is grossly out of step with reality. Even the tolerable upper intake level (UL), which has been set at 2,000 IUs a day, would not be sufficient for a good percentage of people to reach optimum range of this substance. The best plan is to have your doctor check your vitamin D blood levels as you work your dose to optimal levels.

---

85   The tea contains the following ingredients: Milk Thistle, Blessed Thistle, Malva leaves, Marshmallow leaves, Persimmon leaves.

The Six Most Deficient Nutrients besides Vitamin B6, Vitamin C, Iron, and Calcium That Have Gone AWOL in North America!

For many decades now, we have known that the minerals in our soils have been significantly denuded and that many vitamins are processed out of our foods.

I refer to this statement in a research paper from the University of California at Berkeley. According to some of the top scientists in the USA, "steadily and alarmingly, humans have been depleting Earth's soil resources faster than the nutrients can be replenished. If this trajectory does not change, soil erosion, combined with the effects of climate change, will present a huge risk to global food security over the next century."[86]

The article goes on to say that *farming is the main culprit*, which "accelerates erosion and nutrient removal, as the primary game changer in soil health."[87] The answer is much like we recycle paper, glass and aluminum cans, we need to start capturing the nutrients lost from the soil (not just nitrogen, potassium and phosphorus) and put them back.

Until this change takes place, we have four minerals and two vitamins that most people, in fact 95 percent or more, are deficient in. They are **vitamin D, vitamin B12, zinc, iodine, selenium, and magnesium.**

Vitamin D

In the many blood tests I have seen for vitamin D, pretty much everyone in North America who lives in the middle USA and north will be deficient in vit. D unless they supplement. Taking 1,000 IUs a day is barely adequate. In my practice, for all health concerns, I aim for optimal levels for superior health. With this in mind, you will want to ask your family doctor (in Canada—the USA is more lenient with dosages) to prescribe double, triple, or quadruple that dose to even come close to optimal levels. I also take this opportunity to inform you that the glowing benefits of vit. D in research were only shown when vit. D was in optimal range—well into and near the top of the normal range. At the present, the normal range is between 75–250 nmol/L. Blood levels close to 175–225 nmol/L are considered optimal and safe.

---

86 Sarah Yang, "Human security at risk as depletion of soil accelerates, scientists warn," *Berkeley News*, https://1ref.us/1ra (accessed October 28, 2021).
87 Ibid.

What is vitamin D and why is it so important?

Vitamin D is actually not a vitamin but a hormone called "cholecalciferol." It is a type of vitamin D which is made by the skin when exposed to sunlight. It can also be taken as a dietary supplement called vitamin D3. Vitamin D came into prominence when it was discovered that rickets was indeed a deficiency of vitamin D. Ensuing research over the years has propelled the importance of this hormone into great prominence in the past decade.

Adequate vitamin D keeps bones strong by promoting calcium absorption which helps prevent fractures from falls in older people and osteoporosis—a critical problem in those who are middle aged and over. What many don't consider, especially women, is that you need to be looking after your bones when you are in your twenties—not when you are in your forties.

Vitamin D is very important for a healthy immune system and reduces the risk of cancer, especially colon, prostate, and breast cancer. If you are wanting to prevent the flu or colds or other infections, vitamin D is an important consideration. It reduces the risk of diabetes, especially in young people and those living in high altitudes.[88]

It protects against heart disease including high blood pressure and heart failure. It has been shown to reduce the risk of multiple sclerosis (MS), improve respiratory function, and it's used as a preventative measure against seasonal affective disorder (SAD).[89]

There are other not-so-well-known benefits of vitamin D that I have observed as a clinician. One of those is in irritable bowel syndrome (IBS), Crohn's disease, colitis, and other inflammatory conditions. For some reason, if you are low in vitamin D, supplementing with generous levels of vitamin D can result in seemingly miraculous improvements in these challenging diseases.

In my hormone balancing work, vitamin D is again mandatory for my patients because it is a pro-hormone.[90] As such, it helps in the production of many other hormones including the sex hormones estrogen and testosterone. It also helps with overall hormonal balance.

---

88 Editor, "Vitamin D and Diabetes," Diabetes.co.uk, https://1ref.us/1rb (accessed October 28, 2021).
89 "Why Is Vitamin D So Important for Your Health?" HCP Live, https://1ref.us/1rc (accessed October 28, 2021).
90 "Hormone Vitamin D," Hormone Health Network, https://1ref.us/1rd (accessed October 28, 2021).

Is it any wonder why vitamin D should be a staple on everyone's supplement list?

One fact that has emerged is vitamin D deficiency is rampant not only in North America, but worldwide requiring *everyone* to supplement to a certain degree with D3, especially those in the more northern climes.

> *One fact that has emerged is vitamin D deficiency is rampant not only in North America, but worldwide requiring everyone to supplement to a certain degree with D3, especially those in the more northern climes.*

The bottom line is that, for various reasons, people don't or can't get enough sunlight. As I have mentioned earlier, getting out in the fresh air and sunlight is of paramount importance and this just adds another reason why.

However, most are conditioned to think that as a fat-soluble vitamin, they can get all they need for the fall and winter by being out in the summer sun. This is a fallacy I have demonstrated many times by testing vitamin D levels clinically. Stores of vitamin D from the summer may last a month or so into the fall at most and by mid to late fall, without any vitamin D supplementation, the levels will plummet.

I recommend my patients supplement with vitamin D3 drops year-round, increasing the dose in the fall and winter and only lowering it if they are going to get lots of sunlight in the nice weather. Even then, it may not be enough. I cite an example of a friend, who I will call Kathryn, who was suffering from hormonal imbalances and depression. She made a point to get out in the summer sun as much as she could, hoping that would increase her vit. D levels and help alleviate the problem. Her symptoms persisted and so at summer's end, she had her vit. D levels tested. The results were 25 nmol/L (reference range is 75–250 nmol/L), showing desperately low levels! This is just one of many examples that I have observed clinically, where, despite sun exposure, extra supplementation was still required.

If you have brown or black skin, your need for vitamin D is even *greater* than that of Caucasian skin because the protective melanin levels are higher, and so less vitamin D can be produced at the skin level with exposure to the sun. You will need to take extra supplemental vit. D to compensate. Another point to remember is that for superior uptake of vit. D, because it is fat-soluble, it is best taken with a meal which contains fat.

The mystery of vitamin B12

What is very strange about this nutrient, which is classed as a B vitamin, is that while many people test well for B12 on blood tests, many exhibit deficiency symptoms. When we provide them with a patented sublingual form, which is equal to a regular B12 shot, their symptoms improve or go away altogether. I have found this time and time again and have discovered that it is the case with other clinicians as well. The dosage I usually recommend is 1000 IUs once or twice daily between main meals.

It used to be thought that only vegans were susceptible to a B12 deficiency, but that is only partly true. Most vegans can get enough B12 as long as they eat a B12-fortified food each day, such as a fortified nut or soy milk or fortified whole grain product, or take a B12 supplement. It is rare anymore that a vegan would be found severely deficient.

However, not only vegans, but all people in North America are at risk regardless of if they eat a plant-based or a meat-based diet. The elderly are particularly at risk as well as those on metformin (a diabetic medication), those that take long-term antacid medications for reflux, or those that lack or are deficient in an important protein called *intrinsic factor* found in the stomach, which is the second step required for B12 absorption into the blood.

Why is B12 important and what are its deficiency symptoms?

B12 is a nutrient that helps keep the body's nerve and blood cells healthy and assists in making DNA, the genetic material in all cells. Clinical deficiency of B12 can cause one or both of the following types of anemia: *Pernicious anemia* occurs when your immune system mistakenly attacks the stomach cells that produce the abovementioned intrinsic factor resulting in B12 deficiency.

Another type of anemia called *megaloblastic anemia* where red blood cells are larger yet deficient in numbers, can also contribute to fatigue and weakness and nervous system damage which can manifest as numbness, tingling,[91] and reduced sensitivity to pain or pressure.

Feeling tired and weak occurs in this case "because your body doesn't have enough vitamin B12 to make red blood cells, which transport oxygen throughout your body."[92] Megaloblastic anemia can also be a deficiency

---

91   "Vitamin B12," National Institutes of Health, https://1ref.us/1re (accessed October 28, 2021).
92   Helen West, "9 Signs and Symptoms of Vitamin B12 Deficiency," healthline, https://1ref.us/1rf (accessed October 28, 2021).

of folacin, or folic acid, so blood tests should be run to determine which of these two nutrients it is or if it's both.

Other symptoms that I have observed include mild to moderate depression, poor memory, confusion, hallucinations, personality changes, blurred vision, abnormal gait, and sore tongue. Supplementation is almost always sure to correct these deficiency symptoms as long as it has not been too long-term. The best way to supplement B12 is with a good quality sublingual tablet that dissolves under your tongue.

Zinc

Many years ago—1984 to be exact—I completed my PhD dissertation which focused on all the known research and understanding of the function of zinc in nutrition and its purpose in the body.

At the time, it was becoming more and more understood for its significant importance in the human system and what symptoms could result should it be deficient. I made the prediction that, in time, with continued research, zinc might even eclipse iron in importance. I believe that today, nearly forty years later, it has. Certainly, zinc has a significantly greater amount of responsibility in the body than iron and it seems we are learning more and more as time goes on.

With greater and greater knowledge and understanding, this mineral has also been recognized as being more scarce in our soils and foods than ever. In clinical testing with my patients over the years, there has been a demonstrable increase in the number of men, in particular, who show deficiency (often severe), of this important mineral. Why would this seem to affect more men than women?

In men, large amounts of zinc are found in the semen, and with each ejaculation, more zinc is used up from body stores. Zinc is also important for the health of the prostate and the production of prostatic fluid. In addition, it is required for the numerous other functions such as immune system support, cell division, cell-growth, wound healing, providing for the senses of smell and taste, and to facilitate hundreds of enzymatic reactions—to list just a few.

Because of its role in male sexual function, it is postulated that without it there is reduced sexual competency and erectile dysfunction. Indeed, it is involved in the production of two key sex hormones: testosterone and prolactin. In addition to these, it has a role in the metabolism of estrogen and progesterone, together with the prostaglandins, as well as a role in the secretion of insulin. Because of this, it is clear that zinc is also vital for women who are often lacking in this invaluable metal. For women, this too has its impact on hormonal balance and overall well-being.

To correct these often-long-standing deficiencies (which I determine in a simple in-clinic test), it can take months and months. An over-the-counter zinc is almost useless and I employ a highly absorbable form of liquid zinc to make any progress. Second best is to purchase some zinc lozenges at any health food store and suck on them each day. Once you reach an optimal level, men and women over the age of forty should take 20–40 mg of zinc daily for maintenance, prostate health, and hormone balance.

Iodine

Iodine is another mineral that is often deficient over a wide percentage of our North American population. Some estimates are as high as 90 percent and the World Health Organization (WHO) proclaims it the number one prevention of physical disabilities, especially in utero (before birth). In fact, for several years, I conducted lab tests in my clinic for iodine deficiency and I did not find **one single person who was not deficient in iodine.** I gave up testing and put all patients on iodine!

Why would I do that? Well, it just so happens that iodine is the principal raw material the body uses to make thyroxine, the main hormone required by the thyroid gland, which is part of the endocrine system.

Thyroid hormones play a significant role in bone and brain development during pregnancy and infancy. They also aid in both the growth of cells and the repair of damaged cells. Although paying attention to iodine levels is important for everyone, it's absolutely critical for infants and pregnant women.

It is also important to know that this extremely important organ, along with the adrenal glands, are the two main glands in the body responsible for the production of energy. If almost everyone is deficient in iodine, not only does it affect the balance of other endocrine glands (the adrenals in particular), but an under-functioning thyroid (hypothyroid) can cause significant issues in the body.

Let's begin to list the main symptoms of iodine deficiency and I think you will see how broadly this mineral impacts bodily function:

- low energy and fatigue
- weakness
- cold extremities
- brittle, straw-like hair and nails
- dry and scaly skin

- weight gain
- cyst formation—particularly thyroid, breasts, ovaries, and uterus
- prostate concerns for men
- immune system
- constipation
- depression
- low libido (sex drive)
- irregular or heavy periods
- goiter (swelling of the thyroid)

Since it was discovered many decades ago that iodine deficiency was responsible for causing an alarming increase in goiter, iodine was added to salt to ensure that people received supplementary sources of it. Because excess table salt has been labelled as a potential cause for high blood pressure, the use of it has been strongly discouraged and, as a result, we have seen a tremendous rise in hypothyroidism over the past few decades.

Although an under-active thyroid affects both men and women, women seem more susceptible.

Iodine also affords protection in preventing cancers of the breast, ovaries, and uterus in women and the prostate in men.[93] Taking a little iodine each day for your thyroid is among the cheapest health insurance money can buy! I recommend, for maintenance, 150–300 micrograms daily.

Selenium

Here is another crucial trace mineral that is deficient in varying degrees in our population. Deficiencies of selenium can cause infertility in men and women, muscle weakness, fatigue, mental fog, hair loss, and weakened immune system.

Much research into the effects of a deficiency of this mineral has been done in China and has determined that if the lack of this mineral continues long enough and there is exposure to Coxsackievirus, it can cause Keshan disease. Coxsackieviruses are contagious and can cause symptoms ranging from very mild to severe. It is often a cause of the common cold. Keshan disease is a congestive cardiomyopathy which leads to a weakening of the heart and can be fatal. Selenium deficiency also contributes to Kashin-Beck disease which results in atrophy, degeneration, and necrosis of cartilage tissue in the joints.[94]

---

[93] Saeed Kargar, Seyed Mostafa Shiryazdi and Mahdieh Kamali, "Urinary Iodine Concentrations in Cancer Patients," *Asian Pacific Journal of Cancer Prevention* 18 (2017): pp. 819-821.

[94] *Iodine, Selenium Deficiency and Kashin-Beck Disease*, ed. by Victor R. Preedy, Gerard N. Burrow and Ronald Watson (Elsevier Inc, 2009) Comprehensive Handbook of Iodine.

A principal concern for us in North America is not so much the above-mentioned conditions, which are relatively rare here, but compromised immunity. More research needs to be done, but it is generally accepted that adequate selenium can reduce your risk of certain cancers such as prostate, colon, gastrointestinal, lung, and breast and its strong antioxidant properties lend itself to being cardioprotective.[95]

Recent research has also shown selenium to be an antiviral agent. A deficiency will lead to increased viral pathogenesis; therefore, adequate levels of selenium can help to prevent against viral infection.[96]

Although there are trace amounts of this valuable mineral in most vegetables and whole grains, the greatest plant-based source is found in Brazil nuts. Nonetheless, due to a lack of this nutrient in our soils, a selenium supplement daily of 100 micrograms is highly recommended and is excellent and inexpensive health insurance.

> *Recent research has also shown selenium to be an antiviral agent. A deficiency will lead to increased viral pathogenesis; therefore, adequate levels of selenium can help to prevent against viral infection.*

Magnesium

The mineral magnesium is normally quite plentiful in our food supply, but according to ScienceDaily "up to 50 percent of the US population is magnesium deficient."[97] What are the reasons why a mineral that is present in so many foods be so deficient in our Western populations?

Reasons for magnesium deficiency

"Magnesium is needed for more than 300 biochemical reactions in the body. It helps to maintain normal nerve and muscle function, supports a healthy immune system, keeps the heartbeat steady, and helps bones

---

95 Jillian Kubala, "7 Science-Based Health Benefits of Selenium," healthline, https://1ref.us/1rg (accessed October 28, 2021).
96 Melinda Beck, "Selenium as an antiviral agent," Springer Link, https://1ref.us/1rh (accessed October 28, 2021).
97 American Osteopathic Association, "Low magnesium levels make vitamin D ineffective: Up to 50 percent of US population is magnesium deficient," ScienceDaily, https://1ref.us/1ri (accessed October 28, 2021).

remain strong. It also helps adjust blood glucose levels. It aids in the production of energy and protein."[98]

Where things go wrong with this fourth most prolific mineral in the body is due to a number of reasons. First, it is frequently stripped from foods during processing. If a person is eating packaged, processed food, they can easily miss getting adequate daily magnesium. Another cause is stress. Magnesium is a stress mineral and is required in higher amounts when a person is undergoing anxiety, worry, and other mental and emotional upsets. Alcoholism or excess alcohol consumption will also deplete magnesium.

Health problems associated with magnesium loss include diabetes, poor absorption, chronic diarrhea, celiac disease, and hungry bone syndrome.

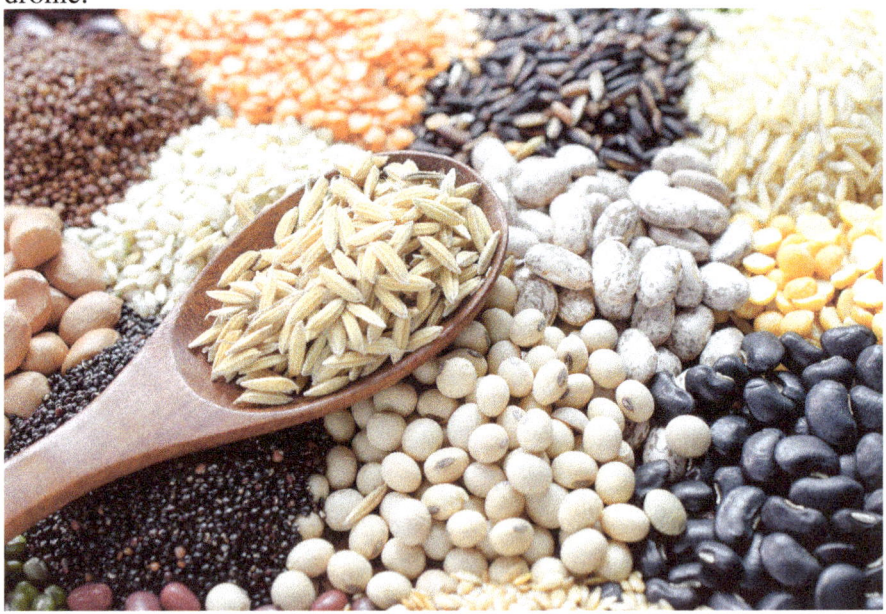

Food sources of magnesium

You will find generous amounts of magnesium in fruits such as bananas, dried apricots, and avocados, nuts such as almonds and cashews, peas and beans (legumes), seeds, soy products like soy flour and tofu, and whole grains such as brown rice and millet.

Choosing to eat a whole-food, plant-based diet will ensure you receive the recommended amounts of magnesium daily. However, if you are under constant stress or suffer from the conditions listed above, it is very

---

[98] "Magnesium in diet," MedlinePlus, https://1ref.us/1rj (accessed October 28, 2021).

important to consider taking extra magnesium in the form of a supplement. I recommend 100–300 mg in divided doses daily. For example, if taking 200 mg, take 100 at breakfast and 100 at bedtime.

Do you have a magnesium deficiency?

Some clear signs of possible magnesium depletion are muscle cramps and twitches, mental disorders such as apathy and a greater risk of depression. It may possibly be linked with anxiety, but more research is needed to see a direct causal connection.

Osteoporosis, which is commonly thought of as a lack of exercise, old age, and a poor intake of vitamins D and K, can also be caused by magnesium deficiency because deficiency lowers the blood levels of calcium, the main building block of bones.[99]

Other signs and symptoms of magnesium deficiency are fatigue, muscle weakness, high blood pressure, severe asthma, and irregular heartbeat.[100] It is important to know that these symptoms could also be indicators of other health disorders and should be checked out by a qualified health practitioner.

One other significant finding about magnesium deficiency that has come to light recently is that vitamin D cannot be metabolized without adequate magnesium levels. Consequently, for the 50 percent or so of Americans who are not getting enough magnesium, their vitamin D is stored and inactive, resulting in them not getting the important vit. D benefits. Furthermore, this situation can increase the calcium and phosphate levels, which may cause vascular calcification if magnesium levels are inadequate to prevent this complication.[101]

These are the basic nutritional supplementation essentials. Of course, depending on the unique needs of the individual, there may be specific or targeted products added. For example, if it is determined that you have adrenal fatigue or a deficiency in digestive enzymes, then appropriate supplementation here will be very helpful. An evaluation by a qualified health professional will be extremely worthwhile to determine an optimal supplement program for you.

---

99 Atli Arnarson, "7 Signs and Symptoms of Magnesium Deficiency," https://1ref.us/1rk (accessed October 28, 2021).
100 Ibid.
101 American Osteopathic Association, "Low magnesium levels make vitamin D ineffective: Up to 50 percent of US population is magnesium deficient," ScienceDaily, https://1ref.us/1ri (accessed October 28, 2021).

You may be inclined to put this off as being too expensive or time-consuming, but investing in your health doesn't cost—it pays. You either pay now or pay much more later!

Extra TRANSFORMational Tip for Supplementation:

Once or twice each week, I take an herbal bowel tonic in the form of a tea or capsule to be sure the bowel is adequately cleansing and not allowing a buildup of toxic waste in what is essentially the sewage system of the body.

This should be done regardless of whether you have constipation or a sluggish bowel or not. This is so very important because the majority of our ills begin in the bowel. A toxic bowel has a profound effect on the rest of the body because of a backup of these impurities into the liver. These toxins are reabsorbed via the bloodstream into the rest of the body. In fact, there are two powerful, proactive measures you can take to keep the burden of toxins in your body at as low a level as possible. One is by taking a daily fiber supplement along with the bowel tonic one to two or more times a week and then every spring and fall undertake a more aggressive bowel/body cleanse. My advice: "Detoxify or die!"

Early on in my recovery (discussed in "Only two years to live!") more than forty years ago, I was fascinated with how natural herbs and nutrition made such an impact on my health and how medications (particularly abuse of antibiotics) gradually destroyed my health. I wanted to learn more and more about how natural and nutritional remedies could be used to actually treat health conditions rather than using drugs, which always had their risks and side effects. I grew up on prescriptions for this and that and, of course, the daily use of over-the-counter drugs for all my respiratory and allergy issues.

My interest was not unfounded, for, as time went on, a whole wide world was opened to me in a myriad of ways, including how endless numbers of ailments could be treated successfully with natural medicine. At the same time, the truth was coming out about the dangers of over-the-counter and prescription drugs. Senior fellow in health policy at George Washington University Medical Center, Thomas Moore, spent six years researching and writing about safety issues surrounding prescription drugs.[102]

---

102 Thomas J. Moore, *Prescription for Disaster* (New York, NY: Simon and Schuster: Rockefeller Center, 1998), pp. 42–56.

He warned in his book entitled *Prescription for Disaster*, which came out in the late 1990s, that in the entire pharmacopeia of medical practice then existing, only four drugs could be considered "safe" and that "adverse reactions to drugs rank as one of the greatest manmade dangers in modern society" with "approximately ... one million severely injured"[103] annually in the United States. Adverse effects of common prescriptions include perforated ulcers, brain damage, addiction, cancer, cardiac arrest, and death.[104]

Even more troubling documentation was tracked in a more recent book, *Death by Medicine*. Here the authors meticulously document that annually in the United States there are an approximate 2,200,000 adverse reactions to prescribed drugs, and 784,000 related to medical prescriptions, administered treatments and interventions. This is a comparable loss of life from 1,568 jumbo jet total fatality crashes. From this we learn that iatrogenic causes (drug or doctor-induced) have taken first place in the leading cause of death in the USA, exceeding the annual death toll from cardiovascular disease, as well as cancer.[105]

It seemed that as I began my practice, recommending the things that I had learned, I was blessed with amazing results, even though I didn't really know what I was doing. I remember my very first patient had been recommended to me by her father who was my insurance agent. She suffered from vicious migraine headaches and I will never forget her words to me as I sat down with her: "I had decided to give the medical profession one year to help me resolve these terrible migraines and if, after one year, I still had them, I would give natural methods a try. So, here I am!" She and I were both thrilled that after about two months she was migraine free. She told the whole town it seems, and my practice started to grow. The last I'd heard, the migraines never came back. She moved out to British Columbia and got a job as—wouldn't you know it—an assistant to a naturopathic physician.

Some months later, a woman whom I shall call Dorothy, came to me with a diagnosis of multiple sclerosis (MS). She had a highly responsible position in the community and by this point she could no longer work. She had heard of me and with great difficulty she made her way into my little office. By this time, we had moved out of the apartment where I had

---

103 Gary Null, Martin Feldman, Debora Rasio and Carolyn Dean, *Death by Medicine*, revised ed. (Mount Jackson, VA: Prakitos Books, 2011), pp. 1–157.
104 Thomas J. Moore, *Prescription for Disaster* (New York, NY: Simon and Schuster: Rockefeller Center, 1998), pp. 42–56.
105 Gary Null, Martin Feldman, Debora Rasio and Carolyn Dean, *Death by Medicine*, revised ed. (Mount Jackson, VA: Prakitos Books, 2011), pp. 1–157.

started my humble little practice and into a larger apartment owned by my parents-in-law. I was no longer the "greenhorn" that I was with my first patient, but MS was the most advanced condition that I had encountered at the time. I still remember how as each month went by, she followed my treatment plan to the letter. By the grace of God, she eventually got better and better until she was able to go back to work full time and she never looked back from there. She is still alive today, some thirty-eight years or so later, and has enjoyed a wonderful, quality life throughout that entire time. It was Dorothy, through her miraculous recovery, that put me on the map. I have never looked back since then either!

The scope of this book does not allow me to go into this area further, much as I would like to. Because of the vast amount of very interesting, fascinating, challenging, unusual, and difficult cases that I have had the privilege to handle over the years, it is my hope that I can devote an entire book on this subject someday soon. Stay tuned!

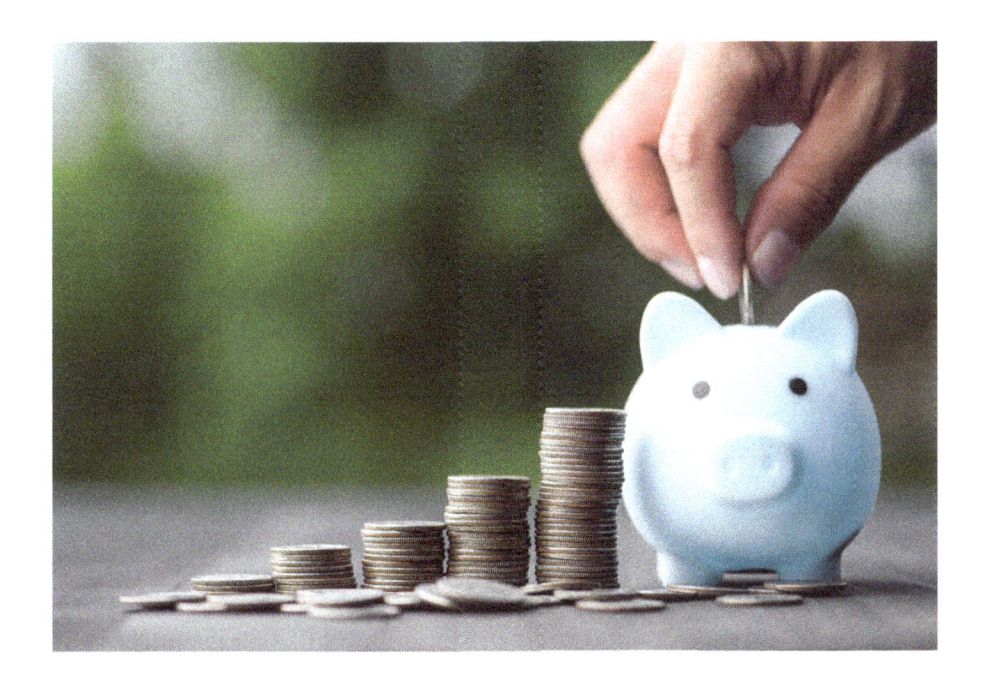

F is for ... Finances

If I were asked what courses should be mandatory in high school, one of them would be a class for students on wise money management! In general, it's not how much you earn but *how much you spend* that is key in this area.

It cannot be overlooked that one of the most challenging and potentially damaging areas of relationships is **finances**. In many domestic disputes, wrangling over the money—or the lack of it—is right at the heart of countless marriage breakdowns.

Scores of people see their only hope as one day winning the lottery and consequently are continually spending their limited resources on all kinds of tickets from the multitude of lotteries available. Yet, statistics tell us that even if one did win the lottery (and those odds are very long—like getting struck dead by lightning or having quadruplets) after five years, 44 percent are broke and after seven years, that figure rises to 70 percent! Odds are if you don't know how to handle money carefully, it will fly the coop. Not recommended for most people.

To be transformed in the area of finances is a topic that can be very complex, but if one follows the general principles found herein, it will go a long way to getting their financial house in order.

So, what are the TRANSFORMational financial practices that can turn your life around in this area?

Here are the basic and simple 7 keys to successfully acquire financial stability and wealth:

1. **Put aside a minimum of 10 percent of your earnings for the Lord and 10 percent for savings.** For those who are wondering how putting this much aside can work, God has asked us to return to Him a tithe of 10 percent (the word "tithe" literally means 10 percent) of our earnings (Mal. 3:10). In my experience and that of many others, following this practice has provided me with much more in return than I have given. God is faithful and His promises are always true. Following all seven keys will demonstrate that we can learn to manage quite well with 80 percent of our earnings.

2. **Control your spending.** Set up a monthly budget for the purpose of helping your savings to grow. Budget enough to cover your necessities and to enjoy some extra worthwhile expenditures as is attainable without spending more than eight-tenths of your earnings.

3. **Put your savings to work.** The 10 percent we put aside each month representing our savings is just the start. The earnings it will make will reap you a fortune. For those who are young (under age thirty-five) the power of compounding interest is something to behold. See the startling example below:

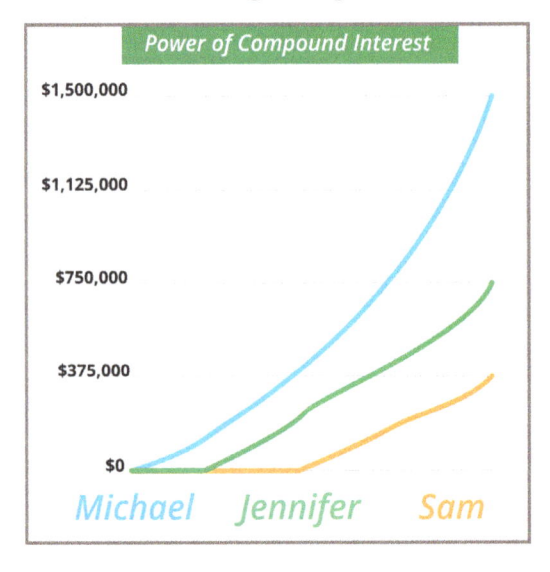

Power of Compound Interest

- $1,500,000
- $1,125,000
- $750,000
- $375,000
- $0

Michael   Jennifer   Sam

Michael saved $1,000 per month from the time he turned twenty-five until he turned thirty-five. Then he stopped saving but left his money in his investment account where it continued to accrue at a 7 percent rate until he retired at age sixty-five.

Jennifer held off and didn't start saving until age thirty-five. She put away $1,000 per month from her thirty-fifth birthday until she turned forty-five. Like Michael, she left the balance in her investment account, where it continued to accrue at a rate of 7 percent until age sixty-five.

Sam didn't get around to investing until age forty-five. Still, he invested $1,000 per month for ten years, halting his savings at age fifty-five. Then he also left his money to accrue at a 7 percent rate until age sixty-five.

Michael, Jennifer, and Sam each saved the same amount—$120,000—over a ten-year period.

Sadly, for Jennifer, and even more so for Sam, their ending balances were dramatically different. However, no matter what your age, it is never too late to start—just keep putting money away each month and don't stop!

SAVER	Totals:
Michael	$1,444,969
Jennifer	$734,549
Sam	$373,407

4. **Protect your investments.** The adage, "A fool and his money are soon parted" rings as true today as it ever did. We must be careful to secure the principal and not risk its loss by the promise of larger returns. Study each investment opportunity, carefully weighing the pros and cons but better by far to consult the wisdom of those experienced in handling money for investment. Ideally it should be a reasonably safe place where it may be accessed if necessary and has a fair rate of return. Let their knowledge protect and help grow your wealth. Before you loan money to anyone, be sure of his/her ability to repay and his/her reputation for doing so.

5. **Own your own home.** As much as possible, you need to purchase your own home rather than rent. With the amount of money you pay in rent every month, you could, instead, be putting it toward a mortgage payment, which is gradually building equity in your home. One of the challenges you may have is coming up with the down payment for a home. This is where you could put your 10 percent that you put aside each month as savings from your earnings. In Canada, there is currently a plan available (**Home Buyers' Plan—HBP**) in which a first-time homebuyer can use pre-tax dollars and apply it as a down payment for a home purchase.

   Another strategy to employ if paying the mortgage, taxes, and utilities is a bit steep, is to **make an apartment in the basement or separate area of the home and rent it out.** The rent that is taken in will partially or even completely defray your expenses and allow you to actually come out ahead financially.

6. **Estate planning.** As you accrue wealth, you may want to be thinking about providing an income for yourself and family during the time when you might like to retire or at the very least slow down a bit. You will also want to have a last will and testament in place to provide for your family and the costs that come with your demise. At as early an age as possible, take out some *life insurance to* protect you and your family against unpaid loans, debts, mortgages, and other financial commitments should something unexpectedly happen to you. There are definitely some excellent insurance products out there today that will give you a lot more scope than in years past. The best advice is to consult with a qualified insurance agent who comes highly recommended.

7. **Increase your earning ability.** Become the best you can be with the strengths with which the Lord has blessed you. Be the most knowledgeable, learned, wise, innovative, dependable in your field—a game changer is the word I like. Be absolutely militant and fanatical in learning and doing all you can to advance in skill in your work so that each week, each month, each year you are so valuable that you are worth more and more to your employer or your business.

Extra TRANSFORMational Tip for Finances:

The Bible says, "[f]or the love of money is a root of all *kinds of* evil" (1 Tim. 6:10). Rather than being a slave to your money, it should be regarded as a servant, ever ready to provide the means to support yourself and your family. The next step is to **find a cause or causes that you can support** not only with your time but also with your money. If you can use your resources to make a difference in the lives of those less fortunate, you have done the work that Christ would have you do. The tithe you return can be used for this if it is promoting God's work, but if you are able to give more, don't stop there. The story is told by the legendary Pastor Henry Feyerabend of a discussion on the topic of tithing amongst a small group traveling by helicopter. One of the group, an extremely wealthy businessman, confessed that he did not tithe 10 percent and hoped that God would forgive him. Now, Pastor Feyerabend was puzzled over this because they were traveling in this very man's own helicopter over numerous large mission projects that he had donated and built with his own funds. He turned to the man and said, "Well, with what I see, you must be awfully close to your 10 percent!" The man replied with a wink, "I keep the 10 percent for myself ... and give the rest away! I hope the Lord will approve!"

More Advanced TRANSFORMational Tips for Finances:

As citizens of whatever country you are from, we all know that taxes, whether it's sales tax, gasoline tax, property tax, federal tax, and death taxes to name a few, can take up a rather large chunk of our income. Although we don't have much choice with a number of taxes which are either built into the prices we pay for things or applied as a percentage of the value of something, there are some exceptions. In Canada, it is good to know that you can exert some control over the biggest taxes you have to pay which are federal, provincial, and estate taxes. These taxes can be significantly modified up or down by the way you arrange your financial affairs.

In his book, *The 10 Secrets Revenue Canada Doesn't Want You to Know*, author and financial planner, David M. Voth, provides a number of strategies that you can employ and that *do* work. It is important, however, that you utilize these strategies with the assistance of a professional, qualified tax advisor. Every individual's financial situation is different and therefore requires a careful approach that should be left to someone who knows how to guide them in their game plan.

Space does not permit me to go into detail on these tips, but I want to briefly mention them so that you can look into it and see if your accountant or financial advisor feels this will be of benefit to you.

1. **Take Maximum Advantage of Your Registered Retirement Savings Plan (RRSP):** As a tax shelter, RRSPs are hard to beat. There are very few of us who would not benefit from this. The following are some tips that are important to know to optimize your RRSP contributions.

   a) Contribute as early in the year as possible.

   b) Contribute anyway and delay the deduction if you are in a low income bracket and don't need to claim the deduction. When you are in a higher income position, you can apply it then.

   c) Put your interest earning investments into your RRSP.

   d) Transfer your retiring allowance or severance pay to your RRSP.

   e) Name your spouse as beneficiary or lose 52 percent of your RRSP.[106]

2. **Open a Tax-Free Savings Account (TFSA):** TFSA is a wonderful gift from the government that you must, if at all possible, take advantage of. You can chunk away up to a certain amount annually with pre-tax income and it's non-taxable if you need to take it out for an important purchase or an emergency.

   If you are married or have a partner, make sure he or she opens one in their name as well. Another benefit is that if you were unable to contribute the maximum in a particular year, you can top it up at any given time retroactive to the time you opened the account.

   To power this up even more, it is worth mentioning that the TFSA can be used in combination with the RRSP and is a great savings vehicle to use if you're looking to save up for a major purchase or rainy-day fund. You can withdraw funds in the future without penalty while having your money grow tax-free.

3. **Earn Dividends Instead of Interest:** Convert your interest earning investments (e.g., GICs and bonds) into dividend earning investments. "You pay less tax on the dividend income than you would

---

106 David M. Voth, *The 10 Secrets Revenue Canada Doesn't Want You to Know* (Saskatoon, SK, CA: Voth Publications, 1996), pp. 20–22.

on an interest payment."[107] If capital is being returned from the original amount invested, you can qualify for capital gains treatment which is also preferable to income tax rates but is more complex than a simple dividend payment.

4. **Use Charitable Giving to Enhance the Recipient's and Your Position:** By giving to religious or needy community organizations or other worthy charities, you can reduce your taxes at the same time. Charitable donations entitle you to earn tax credits. All donations above $200 made during the year earn you a 29 percent federal tax credit. If you are in a higher taxable income bracket, when you add in the effect of the provincial tax, this credit is worth about 50 percent of your donation. At this rate, "for each one dollar you donate, approximately fifty cents comes right back into your pocket."[108]

Example #1: Taxable income up to $200,000

A donor in Alberta with a taxable income of $40,000 donates $700 in 2016. Their tax credit is calculated as the total of the following:

Federal charitable donation tax credit

$30 (15 percent on the first $200)
$145 (29 percent on the remaining $500)
$175 ($30 + $145) is their total tax credit

Provincial charitable donation tax credit

$20 (10 percent on the first $200)
$105 (21 percent on the remaining $500)
$125 ($20 + $105) is their total provincial tax credit
$300 ($175 + $125) is their total charitable donation tax credit for 2016

Example #2: Taxable income over $200,000

A donor in Alberta with a taxable income of $215,000 donates $20,000 in 2016. Their tax credit is calculated as the total of the following:

---

107 Ibid., p. 27.
108 Ibid., pp. 37–38.

Federal charitable donation tax credit

$30 (15 percent on the first $200)
$4,950 (33 percent of $15,000)
which is the lesser of the following:
- the amount by which their total donation exceeds $200 ($19,800)
- the amount by which their taxable income exceeds $200,000 ($15,000). $19,800 − $15,000 = $4,800

$1,392 (29 percent of $4,800) which is the amount of their total donations for the year over $200 that is not eligible for the 33 percent rate above ($19,800 − $15,000)
$6,372 ($30 + $4950 + $1392) is their total federal tax credit

Provincial charitable donation tax credit

$20 (10 percent on the first $200)
$4,158 (21 percent on the remaining $19,800)
$4,178 ($20 + $4,158) is their total provincial tax credit
$10,550 ($6,372 + $4,178) is their total charitable donation tax credit for 2016

5. **Buy an Insurance Tax Shelter:** This is a plan issued by a life insurance company that allows you to deposit any amount of money, and shelter all the growth of the investment from income tax. Your earnings build up tax-free within the plan and the fees that you pay the insurance company annually are less than the income tax you would pay on a non-sheltered investment such as stocks, bonds, GICs, etc.

    Canada Revenue Agency (CRA) "allows insurance companies to issue these plans and maintain their tax-sheltered status as long as they satisfy certain conditions. The insurance company must maintain a minimum amount of insurance on each plan to keep it tax exempt. This insurance however, can and should be low cost decreasing coverage, only enough to keep the plan tax exempt. The amount is based on a Revenue Canada (now called CRA) formula and each plan must meet an annual test."[109]

6. **Start a Small Business:** This may be the best tax shelter of all, especially when it is a home office or business. The tax advantages

are significant, with deductions on all your household expenses, car, and gas expense and much more up to a certain percentage.

A bed and breakfast is one of the best home businesses you can operate in order to create the most significant tax-deductible expenses.

Another idea, as mentioned earlier, is to make a portion of your home into a legal apartment to rent out. If your home is big enough to make a reasonably sized apartment according to guidelines, this can be a great avenue for income. Not only is it a good source of income to help bring down your overhead or put against a mortgage, but there is also a substantial degree of write-offs you can make against your income.

Disclaimer: I am **not** a financial planner or advisor. For your own financial planning or advice, please consult a qualified financial advisor. This is strictly for general informational and educational purposes.

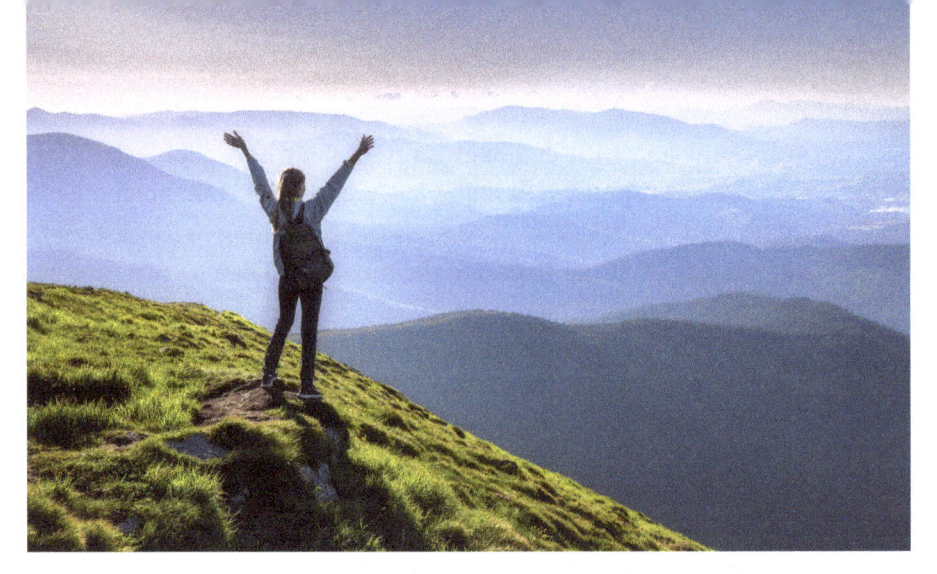

O is for … Outlook

Outlook on life has a much greater, more profound effect on our health than we give it credit for! The Bible is clear on this, for it says in Proverbs 17:22 (ESV), "A joyful heart is good medicine," but goes on with the admonition, "but a crushed spirit dries up the bones."

There is so much on this topic for which countless self-help books have been written. I will attempt to touch on the high points of this grossly underestimated and underrated aspect of our nature. I will also share, at least in part, the incredible effect our thoughts, outlook, and attitude have on the total health of our mind, body, and spirit.

> *An optimistic outlook helps us to get the most out of life. It's essential to health, happiness, and abundance. Outlook is a gift we give to ourselves and our health.*

An optimistic outlook helps us to get the most out of life. It's essential to health, happiness, and abundance. Outlook is a gift we give to ourselves and our health.

A negative outlook turns off the lights of hope, changes love into hate and peace into stress. But a positive outlook does the opposite. It brings hope, ignites love, and sets hearts ablaze. A positive outlook is available through the power of our Creator. Positive is what He made us to be—positive like Himself.

Although many people don't think of this, each of us actually has a choice: to be either positive or negative (pessimistic). Each day you are making that choice ... sometimes even moment by moment. How about *your* attitude? Do you generally have a good or a bad attitude?

A person with an optimistic outlook is the kind of person who doesn't accept failure. It is not an option. He or she searches for solutions and remains committed to the worthy goals they have set.

Do our thoughts shape our life and affect our health? You bet! The Bible says, "For as he thinks in his heart, so is he" (Prov. 23:7). Napoleon Hill, the author of *Think and Grow Rich,* once said, "You can be anything you want to be, if only you believe with sufficient conviction and act in accordance with your faith; for whatever the mind can conceive and believe, the mind can achieve."[110]

What we get stuck on is do we really believe in ourselves? Belief is a choice, and we cement that belief in our minds by repeating it over and over and over. As Henry Ford once said, "Whether you think you can, or you think you can't, you're right."[111]

Often, if you have been drawn to something you are passionate about and decide this is what you want to do, this can be a very powerful way to generate positive inspiration toward believing whether something can or can't be done.

I remember many years ago when I was recovering from my significant illnesses, I began to see the huge potential that the field of natural medicine could offer to humankind. Keep in mind, however, that at that time there were very few, if any, who did this as a profession; yet I was clearly feeling better than any other time in my life. Growing up in the conventional Canadian home, I had *no inkling* that there was a whole "other" type of medicine out there.

So, I enthusiastically plunged ahead with this dream of being a "natural doctor" even though natural health practitioners were almost non-existent at the time. I didn't even give it a second thought. This was what the Lord wanted me to do and so that's what I was going to do!

Not once did I flinch or falter, especially when so many around me said "it can't be done" or "you won't be able to make a living at something like that." I believed in myself. I could see and feel the healing in my body, and I knew there were countless others out there like me who needed help. Forty years so far in full-time practice and tens of thousands of happy, recovered patients later, I can truly say that despite some very tough and discouraging times, I have never looked back. I give God all the

---

110 Napoleon Hill, *Think and Grow Rich* (New York, NY: Fawcett Books, 1987).
111 Henry Ford, "Whether you think you can, or you think you can't—you're right," *Harrisburg Telegraph*: November, 1947.

credit for blessing me with so many miraculous instances of His blessings, mercy, love, and wisdom. I think it is also important to share that my wife was able to stay home the entire time to raise our beautiful family *on one income*, all the while putting our three boys through private elementary, secondary Christian schools, and university. We own a nice but modest home and have a summer home as well right on Georgian Bay, one of the most sought-after freshwater destinations in the world.

There is much more to add, but suffice to say, the Lord has truly blessed me and has rewarded my faith time and time again. When I stop to think about it, which is rarely, it is mildly satisfying and vindicating in a way to know that all the naysayers and dream stealers in my life who said it couldn't be done were wrong.

Was it always easy? Anyone who has been in business for that long knows that it is anything but a cakewalk with the constant ups and downs of the economy. It is especially more so in a country where almost everyone has access to free medical care compared to over 95 percent of my patients who have to pay out-of-pocket for my services.

On top of all that, the practice of natural medicine has been, over the years, viewed with skepticism, cynicism, disbelief, and persecution. I endured the Q word (quackery) more times than I can think and yet all the while I was happily seeing and positively helping those on whom the medical profession had given up!

This is the kind of outlook *you* need in life. First, find your passion and do whatever it takes to make it happen. Don't let those dream stealers try to bring you down to their level. Most of the time, they have settled for a mediocre life of unhappiness, drudgery, and a deep dissatisfaction with their lot in life. They often have an underlying desire to discourage you from being successful while doing something you love. At the very least, it is better to be poor and happy than well-off and miserable.

Someone who believes in him or herself will need to have an unrelenting resolve that will weather the ups and downs, the storms, the errors in judgment, the mistakes and failures on their journey. These challenges will most assuredly attend their efforts, so it is important to know that anyone who has been blessed with any measure of success will have traveled down that rocky road.

I am so inspired and encouraged by a quote attributed to Calvin Coolidge, the thirtieth president of the United States. I have framed it and it has hung on the wall in my office for many years now.

Press On

"Nothing in the world can take the place of persistence.

Talent will not; nothing is more common than unsuccessful men with talent.

Genius will not; unrewarded genius is almost a proverb.

Education will not; the world is full of educated derelicts.

Persistence and determination alone are omnipotent."[112]

Be an Optimist by Counting Your Blessings

Start shaping your day and your life by choosing to think positively. "Optimists count their blessings. Pessimists count their burdens."[113]

In his book, *Learned Optimism*, Dr. Martin Seligman states that "becoming an optimist consists not of learning to be more selfish and self-assertive, and to present yourself to others in overbearing ways, but simply of learning a set of skills about how to talk to yourself when you suffer a personal defeat."[114] As your optimism improves, you will be able to have a heart-to-heart with yourself and view setbacks from a more positive perspective ... a growing experience, if you like. This technique has become known as cognitive therapy.

Deal with Your Depression Naturally

When we are not optimistic, but focus on the negative, it can lead to depression. In the USA alone, depression affects 19 million and worldwide about 200 million people. This is a huge problem and accounts for among the most highly prescribed medications. However, cognitive therapy can be of great value in helping depression. This helps people be more optimistic and prevent relapses because they acquire a skill they can use again and again, thus reducing reliance on drugs or doctors. "Drugs relieve depression, but only temporarily; unlike cognitive therapy, drugs fail to change the underlying pessimism which is at the root of the problem."[115]

---

112   Fred R. Shapiro, *The Yale Book of Quotations* (New Haven, CT: Yale University Press, 2006), p. 173.
113   Creation Health: God's 8 Principles for living Life to the Fullest, ed. Robyn Edgerton (Florida Hospital Mission Development, 2012), p. 201.
114   Martin Seligman, *Learned Optimism* (New York, NY: Picket Books, 1998), p. 207.
115   Ibid., p .81.

Many are pessimistic because they do not have a vision for themselves or their future. They don't feel they have a genuine purpose and may feel they are drifting aimlessly. A good vision means that they have meaning and purpose in everything they do. It means they have a positive outlook. A vision is a dream in action. Optimists have a dream. They hold onto that dream when passing through life's dark valleys. They will live and die for their vision.

I encourage each one of you to embrace the vision which is at the very core of the *National Geographic Magazine* and how they represent themselves: "Celebrate What's Right With The World!"[116] A person with an optimistic outlook is the kind of person who indeed celebrates what's right with the world. Having and maintaining this kind of attitude is a powerful, life-shaping force. This is the kind of person whose life is filled with peace and joy because of their implicit trust in God. The result is a cheerful spirit that plays a vital role in creating whole-person wellness.

Explanatory Styles

It is here then that I will introduce what is called "explanatory styles." People who generally tend to <u>blame themselves</u> for negative events believe that such events will <u>continue indefinitely</u>. They let these events affect many aspects of their lives and they display what is called a <u>pessimistic explanatory style</u>. Conversely, in an optimistic explanatory style, uncontrollable negative events are attributed to external rather than internal causes; unstable rather than stable causes; and specific rather than global causes. An optimistic explanatory style is saying "no" to the three *P*'s. In the example below, John has applied for a very desirable job; however, he did not get the job. Here is how his optimistic explanatory style helped him through this:

1. It's not **p**ersonal— "I didn't get the job because they disliked me; they were able to find a more qualified candidate."
2. It's not **p**ermanent— "If I keep trying, I will find another job."
3. It's not **p**ervasive— "I may not be qualified for this job, but I am certainly qualified for others."

The pattern of someone with a pessimistic explanatory style is one who tends to analyze (often overanalyzing) why things go wrong in their lives. Overall, a pessimist feels that he or she doesn't have control over the

---

116 *Creation Health: God's 8 Principles for living Life to the Fullest*, ed. Robyn Edgerton (Florida Hospital Mission Development, 2012), p. 192.

events of his or her life. Often you will hear a pessimist defend their style by saying that they are just being "realistic" or that they are a "realist." Much of the time, unfortunately, this leads to depression.

At the same time, they tend to under-analyze the good things that are happening in their lives—often taking them for granted. The analysis of good things puts us in touch with the pleasures, successes, positive events, and blessings that are in all our lives. It helps us to focus on the positive, to celebrate what's right with the world! It helps us develop an optimistic explanatory style.

So, take a moment each day and write down the good things that are happening in your life and dwell on them only.

Moving from Pain to Power

As you are celebrating the good things that are going on in your journey, it is also important to do an inventory of what words and expressions you are saying, not only to yourself but also in the presence of others. The following is a series of statements that we often find ourselves saying. Next to these statements are alternative expressions which are effectual in inculcating the positive and affirmative direction we need to be reinforcing in our psyche:

Negative and weak expression	Positive and affirming expression
I can't	I won't
I should	I could
It's not my fault	I'm totally responsible
It's a problem	It's an opportunity
I'm never satisfied	I want to learn and grow
Life's a struggle	Life's an adventure
I hope	I know
If only	Next time
What will I do?	I know I can handle it
It's terrible	It's a learning experience

The Five Truths about Fear

For most of us, our outlook may be marred by fears, either real or imagined. It is a fact that most of our fears, perhaps even as high as 90 percent or more, never actually turn out to be true.[117]

When faced with fear, I often remind myself of the FEAR acronym: **F**alse **E**vidence **A**ppearing **R**eal. This serves to help me take a minute and decompress with the repetition of this assertion in my mind.

When we approach the subject of fear, it is of value, I believe, to also be aware of the five truths about fear:

1. The fear will never go away as long as I continue to grow.
2. The only way to get rid of the fear of doing something is to go out ... and do it. Action cures fear. "Now" is the magic word for success.
3. The only way to feel better about *myself* is to go out ... and do it.
4. Not only am I going to experience fear whenever I'm on unfamiliar territory, but so is everyone else.
5. Pushing through fear is less frightening than living with the underlying fear that comes from a feeling of helplessness.

Have an Attitude of Gratitude

Another important part of your outlook on life is the expression of gratitude for whatever you have.

Let's look at what some studies have found that were part of the "Research Project on Gratitude and Thanksgiving." Researchers examined **four** areas related to gratefulness.[118]

In the area of **overall well-being**, grateful people reported higher levels of positive emotions, life satisfaction, vitality, and optimism, and lower levels of depression and stress. The grateful disposition appears to enhance pleasant-feeling states more than it diminishes unpleasant emotions. The researchers found that grateful people do not deny or ignore the negative aspects of life.

In the area of **pro-sociality**, individuals with a strong disposition toward gratitude have the capacity to be empathetic and take the perspective of

---

117 Sarah Fielding, "New Study Shows 91 Percent of Fears Don't Come True," BestLife, https://1ref.us/1rl (accessed October 28, 2021).
118 M. E. McCullough, R. A. Emmons, and J. Tsang, "The Grateful Disposition: A Conceptual and Empirical Topography," *Journal of Personality and Social Psychology* 82 (2002): pp. 112–127.

others. They are rated as more helpful and more generous by people in their social networks.

In the area of **spirituality**, the researchers also found that those who regularly attend religious services and engage in religious activities such as prayer and reading religious material, are more likely to be grateful. Grateful people are more likely to have a knowledge, belief, and understanding of the interconnectedness of all life and feel a commitment and responsibility to others.

In the area of **materialism**, grateful people placed less importance on material goods and were more likely to share their possessions with others. They were less likely to judge their own and others' success in terms of the number of possessions accumulated, and they were less envious of others.

Many years prior to these studies, gifted Christian writer Ellen G. White wrote, "Nothing tends more to promote health of body and of soul than does a spirit of gratitude and praise." [119]

At least once each day, purposefully express your gratitude to others through one or more of the following: words of thanks, a handwritten (yes handwritten) thank you note, a letter thanking someone for their positive impact on your life (be sure to list specifics), or an email thanking someone for something they have done. As we recommended in the chapter on "Rest," before you go to bed each night, thank God for at least three things that you are grateful for and sleep in peace, joy, and contentment!

Attitude

Well-known Christian radio broadcaster, theologian, pastor, and author, Charles Swindoll, wrote in his famous quote on Attitude:

> Attitude, to me, is more important than facts.
>
> It is more important than the past, than education, money, circumstances, than failures and successes, than what other people think, say, or do.
>
> It is more important than appearance, ability, or skill.
>
> It will make or break a business, a home, a friendship, an organization.[120]

---

119   Ellen G. White, *The Ministry of Healing* (Mountain View, CA: Pacific Press, 1905), p. 251.
120   Charles R. Swindoll, goodreads, https://1ref.us/1rm (accessed October 28, 2021).

He goes on to say that despite all that happens in life, the only thing that we can do is play on the one thing we have and that is our attitude. "Life is **ten percent what happens to me and ninety percent how I react to it**."[121]

"We need a daily checkup from the neck up to avoid stinkin' thinkin' which ultimately leads to hardening of the attitudes."[122]
—Zig Ziglar

Attitude determines how a person views their own health. For instance, according to several studies done over the past few years, the answer people give to this simple question—For your age, would you say, in general, that your health is excellent, good, fair, poor, or bad?—is a better predictor of who will live or die over the next ten years than are in-depth physical examinations and extensive laboratory tests.[123]

People who self-rated their health as "poor" were up to six times more likely to die earlier than those who rated themselves in "excellent" health.[124] The results of this study done by researchers of Rutgers and Yale Medical School are consistent with the results of five other large studies that involved more than 23,000 people ranging in ages from 19 to 94.[125]

Mental Imagery

To take this one step further, studies also show that using your mind to imagine the body healing itself can aid the healing process.[126] This is referred to as imagery. An example might be imagining your immune system's cells attacking cancer cells. In this situation, you are imagining that your body is working in a certain way and, therefore, it does work that way. A literature review on imagery shows that this method can also help athletes increase performance, deal with anxiety, chronic and acute pain and rehabilitation from injury and stress.[127] Of course, this doesn't just apply to athletes but to anyone who employs this valuable technique.

---

121 Lou Holtz, goodreads, https://1ref.us/1rn (accessed November 1, 2021).
122 "Zig Ziglar Quotable Quote," goodreads, https://1ref.us/1ro (accessed November 1, 2021).
123 Ellen L. Idler and Stanislav Karl, "Health perceptions and survival: do global evaluations of health status really predict mortality?" *Journal of Gerontology* 46 (1991): pp. S55–S65.
124 Ibid.
125 *Creation Health: God's 8 Principles for living Life to the Fullest*, ed. Robyn Edgerton (Florida Hospital Mission Development, 2012), p. 190.
126 Larry Dossey, *Meaning and Medicine: Lessons from a Doctor's Tales of Breakthrough and Healing* (New York, NY: Bantam Books, 1991), p. 16.
127 "Mental Imagery," Physiopedia, https://1ref.us/1rp (accessed November 1, 2021).

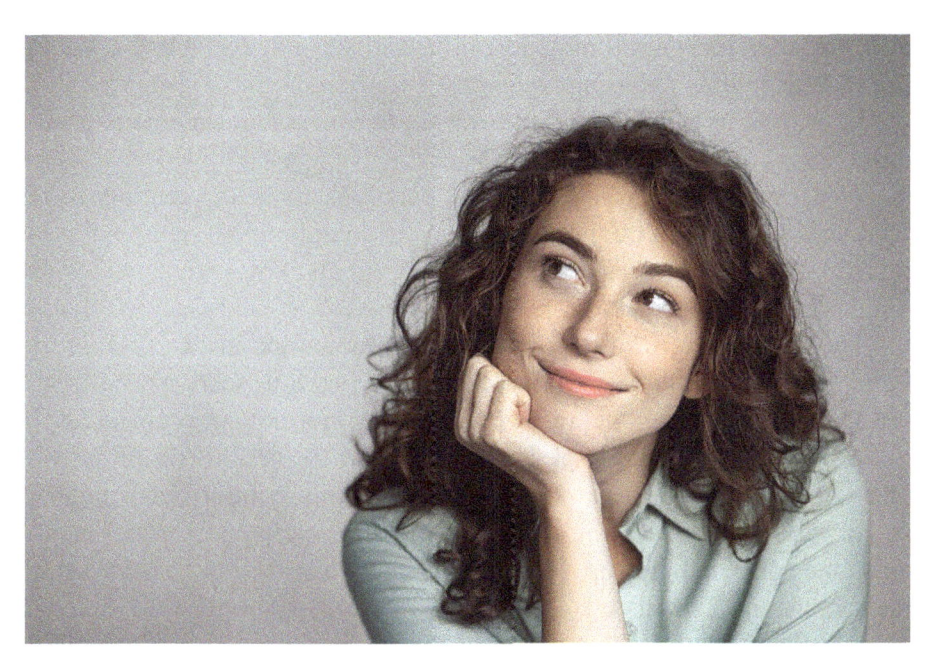

God has given us such a wonderful and powerful gift in our imagination and the ability to envision how things can be accomplished or created. From the Olympic diver who rehearses over and over in his or her mind every intricate move of their dive perfectly before the competition to the neurosurgeon who practices in his mind the entire surgical procedure before he performs his complex surgeries, we too can use this gift of God to accomplish great things.

Each of us, by becoming an optimist and implementing a positive outlook on life, can improve and strengthen our health. By practicing an optimistic outlook, we can actually increase the body's cells that fight off disease. Isn't it amazing that something as simple as choosing to be positive boosts health? This is a wonderful gift from God that we in turn **can give to ourselves.**

According to Herbert Benson in his book, *Timeless Healing: The Power and Biology of Belief*, it has been shown that there is a vital link between religious faith and health.[128] The benefits include improved general health, increased survival; reduced alcohol, cigarette, and drug use; reduced general and death anxiety, reduced depression and hostility; reduced blood pressure; and improved quality of life for patients with cancer and heart disease, and improved psychological symptoms including adjusting and coping. The benefits also include an increase in life and marital satisfac-

---

128 Herbert Benson and Marg Stark, *Timeless Healing: The Power and Biology of Belief* (New York, NY: Fireside (Scribner), 1997), p. 352ff.

tion, and increased well-being, altruism, and self-esteem. Wow! I would call that more than just fringe benefits!

Let's look at a couple of amazing studies on optimism versus pessimism.

This first study was based on 19,781 person-years of observations from current vital status of medical patients who completed an optimism/pessimism scale 30 years earlier. Of the 839 patients, 124 were classified as optimistic, 518 as mixed, and 197 as pessimistic.

Thirty years later the research showed that an optimistic explanatory style (for definition of explanatory styles, see previous section) was associated with a 50 percent decrease in the risk of mortality or early death.[129]

Another good example of mind over matter is the illustration of two oncologists who were discussing papers they were going to present that day at the national meeting of the American Society of Clinical Oncology. One of the physicians was amazed that, while they both were using the same drugs, he was only getting a 22 percent response rate, and his colleague was getting a 74 percent response rate! "That is unheard of for metastatic lung cancer," he said. "How do you do it, Bob?"

The other responded, "We're both using Etoposide, Platinol, Oncovin, and Hydroxyurea. You call yours EPOH. I tell my patients I'm giving them HOPE! Sure, I tell them this is experimental, and we go over the long list of side effects together. But I emphasize that <u>we have a chance</u>."[130]

"A cheerful heart is good medicine" Proverbs 17:22, NLT.

Did you know that laughter is good for our outlook and heart? In fact, researchers found that laughter "actually increases blood flow in the body, proving right the old adage that laughter is the best medicine, at least when it comes to the heart."[131] Doctors at the University of Maryland measured blood flow in twenty healthy men and women before and after watching fifteen- to thirty-minute clips of funny and stressful movies. "While laughing, 19 of the subjects increased healthy blood flow by an average of 22 percent. And comparing the amused and stressful states

---

[129] Toshihiko Maruta, Robert C. Colligan, Michael Malinchoc and Kenneth P. Offord, "Optimists versus Pessimists: Survival Rate Among Patients over a 30-Year Period," Mayo Clinic Proceedings 75 (2000): pp. 140–143.
[130] Norman Cousins, *Head First: The Biology of Hope* (New York, NY: E.P. Dutton, 1989), p. 99, emphasis supplied.
[131] David Biello, "Laughter Proves Good Medicine for Heart," *Scientific American*, https://1ref.us/1rq (accessed November 1, 2021).

brought on by film clips, more than 50 percent more blood flowed when laughing."[132]

One of the most famous illustrations of laughter and healing is that of *Saturday Review* editor Norman Cousins. After a stressful trip to cold-war Russia in 1964, he developed ankylosing spondylitis, a debilitating disease which confined him to bed. He was admitted to the hospital for tests and treatments, but his condition deteriorated and he was told he had little chance of surviving.

Cousins developed a recovery program which incorporated mega doses of vitamin C, along with a positive attitude, love, faith, hope, and laughter induced by Marx Brothers films. "I made the joyous discovery that ten minutes of genuine belly laughter had an anesthetic effect and would give me at least two hours of pain-free sleep,"[133] he reported. After a couple hours, when the pain started to creep back, he would play more of the movie and often he would be pain free again for a time. "When the pain-killing effect of the laughter wore off, we would switch on the movie again and not infrequently, it would lead to another pain-free interval." Slowly, Cousins made a good recovery and lived twenty-six years after the diagnosis of his illness![134]

In an article written by Rod A. Martin, he tackles the question regarding whether children laugh more than adults do. His conclusion, based on various studies, was that children did not necessarily laugh more than adults as many do think. The real determining factor from childhood through to adulthood is how much time during the day we are socially interacting with others.[135] Our next chapter on Relationships will then be important in helping us to work more laughter and fun into our day.

May we make a conscious choice to see the brighter side of life and laugh more often.

When we choose to see the fun and humor in life, we are more optimistic and feel better because of humor's healing effects.

Without having a vision/purpose/mission in life, it's difficult to live life to the fullest because life will become vague and confusing—a wandering generality of sorts, if you will. Vision brings clarity, power, and energy.

---

132 Ibid.
133 Don Colburn, "Norman Cousins, Still Laughing," *The Washington Post*, October 21, 1986.
134 Norman Cousins, *Anatomy of An Illness as Perceived by the Patient: Reflections on Healing and Regeneration* (New York, NY: Norton Publishing, 1979), p. 192.
135 Rod A. Martin, "Do Children Laugh Much More Often than Adults Do?" Association for Applied and Therapeutic Humor, https://1ref.us/1rr (accessed November 1, 2021).

What sentence do you see in this string of letters?

Opportunityisnowhere

"Opportunity is nowhere" or "opportunity is now here?"[136] What you see is what you get!

We can choose to live with a positive vision for our life starting today. It all begins in our minds ….

"You must constantly ask yourself these questions: Who am I around? What are they doing to me? What have they got me reading? What have they got me saying? Where do they have me going? What do they have me thinking? And most important, what do they have me becoming? Then ask yourself the big question: Is that okay?"[137]

Here is another consideration along these lines. Because our thoughts shape who we are, it is vitally important that we choose carefully what we allow to enter our minds, because "[b]y beholding we become changed."[138] It is important for us to think about what we are feeding our minds through TV, movies, books, radio, and the internet.

Too often we go by the maxim, "I won't believe it until I see it." The way it really works is, "I won't see it until I believe it!" A vision or a goal must first be created in the mind. We need to believe it and see it in our mind. Then with a positive attitude and a plan to implement the goal, it can come into being … many times, in ways that appear nothing short of miraculous.

---

136 *Creation Health: God's 8 Principles for living Life to the Fullest*, ed. Robyn Edgerton (Florida Hospital Mission Development, 2012), p. 190.
137 Jim Rohn, *The Treasury of Quotes* (Southlake, TX: Jim Rohn International, 2006), p. 65.
138 Ellen G. White, *The Adventist Home* (Hagerstown, MD: Review and Herald, 1952), p. 330.

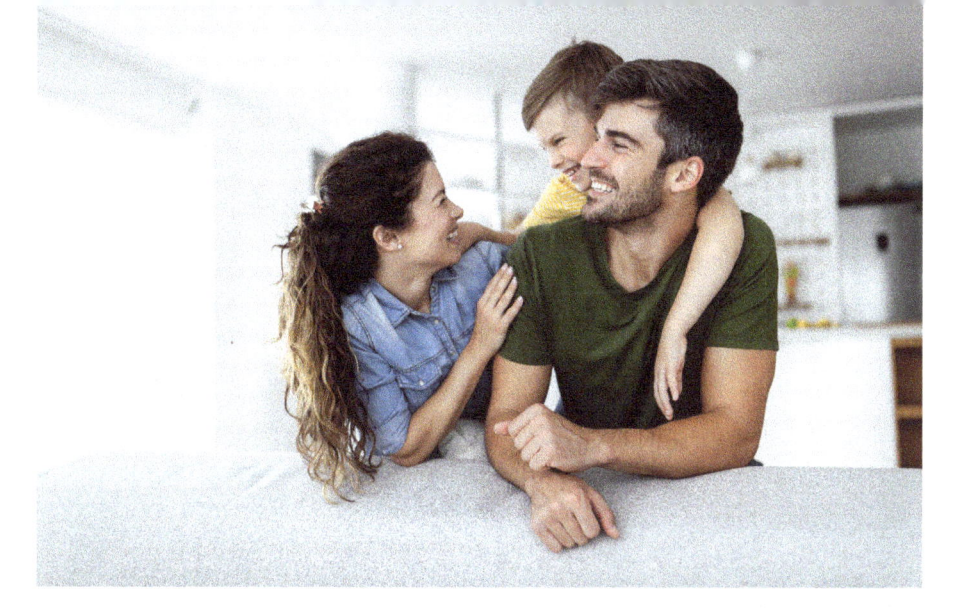

R is for … Relationships

"Iron sharpens iron, and one man sharpens another" (Prov. 27:17, ESV).

Dr. Dean Ornish, in his book, *Love and Survival: The Scientific Basis for the Healing Power of Intimacy,* writes that "I'm not aware of any other factor in medicine—not diet, not smoking, not exercise, not stress, not genetics, not drugs, not surgery—that has a greater impact on our quality of life, incidence of illness, and the premature death from all causes than does love and intimacy."[139]

Being in love with or feeling love from someone can have profound health benefits. "Scientific studies have shown that being in love causes our body to release feel-good hormones and neuro-chemicals that trigger specific, positive reactions. Levels of dopamine, adrenaline and norepinephrine increase when people are in love."[140] The power of love is noted by Dr. Bernie Siegel, Yale physician and author of the best-selling book, *Love, Medicine and Miracles*: "Unconditional love is the most powerful stimulant of the immune system. The truth is love heals."[141]

The Alameda County Study is considered by many as the definitive study on social support and the risk of death. In fact, it is one of the most

---

139 Dean Ornish, *Love and Survival: The Scientific Basis for the Healing Power of Intimacy* (New York, NY: HarperCollins, 1998), pp. 2–3.
140 "Why is love so important?" *The Economic Times*, https://1ref.us/1rs (accessed November 1, 2021).
141 *Creation Health: God's 8 Principles for living Life to the Fullest*, ed. Robyn Edgerton (Florida Hospital Mission Development, 2012), p. 159.

quoted studies in the field of health.[142] This study, which dealt with more than 7,000 people followed for forty years, showed the following:

- People classified as lonely and isolated had three times higher mortality rates
- People with many social contacts had the lowest mortality rates
- The amount of social support was the best predictor of good health

Many other similar large-scale studies have been conducted. And the results? They're the same—those who lacked social ties had an increased risk of dying from coronary heart disease, stroke, cancer, respiratory diseases, gastrointestinal diseases, and all other causes of death.[143]

What do we mean by relationships? Well, it could be with a spouse, a close-knit family, a cherished pet, a good network of friends, a church, or other group affiliations. All of these can have a positive and powerful effect on wellness.

What is it about interpersonal relationships and social connectedness that create such a wonderful benefit to our well-being? For one thing, there is the touch factor, which many studies have proven to be a simple but powerful way of stimulating healthy function. Touch can bring about emotional balance and improved health through its primary conveyance of compassion. In fact, Dacher Keltner, who has done much research on touch over the years has found "that people can not only identify love, gratitude, and compassion from touches but can differentiate between those kinds of touch, something people haven't done as well in studies of facial and vocal communication."[144]

It is interesting to mention at this point how different cultures are more touch-friendly and others are more touch-deprived. One of Dr. Keltner's favorite examples of this was a study from the 1960s by pioneering psychologist Sidney Jourard. Studying friends in conversation together in different parts of the world, there was a vast difference in the amount of touch during those conversations. For example, "[i]n England, the two friends touched each other zero times. In the United States, in bursts of enthusiasm, we touched each other twice …. France, the number shot up to 110 times per hour. And in Puerto Rico, those friends touched each other 180 times!"[145] Here in the Western world, we would do well to learn

---

142 Ibid., p. 160.
143 Ibid.
144 Dacher Keltner, "Hands On Research: The Science of Touch," *Greater Good Magazine*, https://1ref.us/1rt (accessed November 1, 2021).
145 Ibid.

from our French and Latino friends how more touch could positively enhance our relationships.

Seeing the marvelous, positive effect a domestic animal has on people has prompted many professionals involved in counseling clients with emotional and mental stress, depression, anxiety, anger, loneliness, and isolation to encourage bringing a pet into the home or facility where they live.

A study done some years ago in 1991 demonstrates very well why and how this can be so effective. Forty-five adult women were observed by measuring physiological response to stress when in the presence of a friend or a pet or neither. Blood pressure reactivity was recorded and, interestingly enough, the physiological reactivity as expressed in blood pressure was lower in the pet and control group.[146] The conclusion was clear that, unlike a friend who may be considered as being judgmental, the pet provided the unconditional love that is more reassuring and supportive emotionally.

For those of you who are married, you earn extra health points provided your relationship is healthy and loving. Many studies have shown that married individuals live longer, with lower mortality for almost every major cause of death, than those who are single, separated, widowed, or divorced.[147] One of the best anti-aging factors is found in a warm relationship with a spouse.

In one study, a team of researchers found that over 2,800 Dutch citizens, ages fifty-five to eighty-five were positively affected by loving relationships. "Specifically, they found that those who perceived themselves as being surrounded by a loving, supportive circle of friends decreased their death rate by approximately half when compared with those who did not feel the close social support. Another study found that older individuals who perceived their social support as impaired were 340% more likely to die prematurely from all causes.[148]

Quality of Our Relationships

The quality of our relationships matter. One study of midlife women showed that those in highly satisfying marriages and marital-type relationships had a lower risk for cardiovascular disease compared with those in less satisfying marriages. Another interesting study found that couples having a nasty disagreement or prolonged spat actually showed signs of

---

[146] Karen M. Allen, Jim Blascovich, Joe Tomaka, Robert M. Kelsey. "Presence of human friends and pet dogs as moderators of autonomic responses to stress in women," *Journal of Personality and Social Psychology*, Vol. 61, Issue 4 (1991): pp. 582–589.
[147] *Creation Health: God's 8 Principles for living Life to the Fullest*, ed. Robyn Edgerton (Florida Hospital Mission Development, 2012), p. 164.
[148] Ibid., p. 165.

reduced immunity. Other studies have linked disappointing or negative interactions with family and friends with poorer health.[149]

The Three Fundamentals of Strong Relationships

It might be good to discuss what the basic fundamentals are in creating strong relationships in our lives. For most adults, the marriage relationship will be the most important place to focus because marriage is the basis of the family unit, the foundation of society. These principles can also be applied in *any* relationship where there is a need to go deeper, to forge lasting and meaningful associations, rather than ones that are just casual or superficial.

According to Meredith Hansen, PsyD, a psychologist and relationship expert, all strong relationships have three things in common: **trust, commitment, and vulnerability**. "Trust allows a couple to know that their partner is there for them, truly cares about them, is coming from a good place, and supports them,"[150] she said.

Developing Trust

In our marriage, which is now well over forty years, Erika and I have developed a habit of communicating and discussing *everything* that we are doing separately or together. If I am going out somewhere or will be delayed, I will leave a note or a text or make a phone call to be sure that she knows where I am and when I expect to be back. If Erika has a meeting to attend or wants to go to a concert either together or with a friend; if she wants to invite friends over or plans an event with family, she discusses it with me first, especially before committing me or us to a function or some other matter.

If you have a habit of saying something and then flip-flopping or even saying something completely different, that does not bode well for establishing trust. As I always said to my kids, "Say what you mean and mean what you say."

It may appear to some that having to always be on your partner's radar would be undesirable. Rather than feeling stifled, trapped, or imprisoned in our relationship, however, I feel it is liberating. To be accountable to someone you love is no hardship. This is especially true when you know

---

149 "The health benefits of strong relationships," Harvard Health Publishing, Harvard Medical School, https://1ref.us/1ru (accessed November 1, 2021).
150 Margarita Tartakovsky, "3 Keys to a Strong Relationship," https://1ref.us/1rv (accessed November 1, 2021).

they care about you and want to be sure you are okay, and you feel the same about them.

Being sure to discuss upcoming plans for social get-togethers, shopping, vacations, appointments, and many other daily and weekly tasks and future items is so very important. It develops communication which is a critical factor in building trust in a relationship.

When we are both in the habit of bringing forward the things that we would like or need to do, then there is the opportunity for us to discuss together whether or not I, or she, would agree with the proposal. We work out when we would go, who would go (perhaps one or both of us, or with others), and other details. This valuable exercise makes for a much smoother, more harmonious relationship, with less chance of misunderstanding or upset.

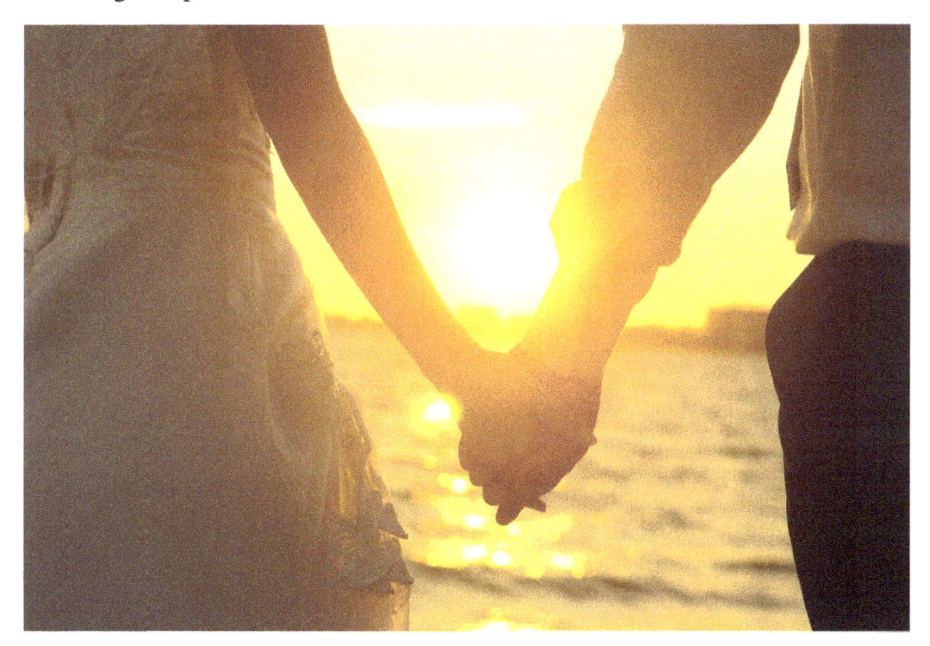

Commitment

When you are developing a new relationship or a veteran of more than four decades like myself, in addition to trust, you will want to display a position of commitment, no matter what the situation may be. In an argument or disagreement or in relationships with other people, either at work or socially, you must both show that your first and foremost concern is to be committed or faithful to the other person. You need to be sure that your spouse knows that you are committed to the relationship and that, come what may, you are both "in this together."

Don't forget that commitment grows as you spend quality time together. That may mean going out on regular "dates" or something just as simple as preparing the meal, or cleaning up the dishes, or folding the laundry together. Have a picture of your spouse on your desk at work, have a playlist of songs that brings back strong memories of your partner, celebrate your wedding anniversary by going through your wedding pictures and/or videos. You must put effort into making these things happen if you want your relationship to last.

Allowing Yourself to be Vulnerable

In a strong relationship, you want to come to a place where you can be genuine, where you can be your real self with your spouse or friend. It comes down to sharing your feelings, not your thoughts. For example, instead of pointing the finger and saying, "You didn't remember my birthday" or "You don't seem to have time for me anymore," it is better to explain, "I feel sad and disappointed that you forgot my birthday" or "It really hurts that you don't find time for me in your busy schedule."

"Vulnerability requires trust and safety in the relationship, but if you can truly make the effort to reveal your softer side, then you'll continue [to] grow closer as a couple," Hansen said. [151]

Growing a strong relationship requires spending a little effort each day in these three important areas (trust, commitment, and vulnerability). In my marriage, I make an effort to kiss my wife in the morning, to exercise touch (which I will expand on later), send love texts, leave an affectionate note where she will see it, make eye contact, share my feelings, goals, and dreams, unplug at our meals together, share family news, listen with my full attention as much as I can, and hear about her latest successes or challenges, her happiness and so on.

What is the Most Important Value a Woman Looks For?

If a person could come up with one word that would most describe what a woman needs to have in a fulfilling and successful relationship, what might that be? Guys, if we really knew the answer to that question, it would be revolutionary, wouldn't it?

Well, I think that word would be … SAFETY … to feel safe mentally, emotionally, physically, spiritually, financially, sexually, and socially with her husband. Feeling *connected and protected* is an important part of the

---
151 Ibid.

safety she wants to feel. Does he keep his promises? Is he trustworthy? Does he give me his undivided energy and attention?

What about the men? What is the highest value of the masculine, gals? The answer is FREEDOM, something which is of critical importance to your male counterpart. This is freedom mentally, emotionally, physically, spiritually, and financially. This, of course, is easier said than done, but the woman who gets this, is rewarded with a husband who is happy, content, and much less likely to roam. He craves appreciation and trust—to be affirmed in his role as the provider and protector in the relationship.

Helper's High

"'It is more blessed to give than to receive'" (Acts 20:35). These words of wisdom spoken by Jesus Christ are proven to be true today by research. "One study showed that what older adults contributed to their social network had more to do with their health than what they received from it."[152]

More study on this interesting phenomena revealed that "95% of those who had regular personal contact with the individuals whom they helped, were blessed with a feel-good sensation which became known as the 'helper's high.'"[153] Another study's participants commented on "the endurance of the glow," or the helper's high. Amazingly, of those who commented, most say that the glow kept returning when they remembered helping. Volunteering is a blessing that "keeps on giving" back to the giver."[154]

Extra TRANSFORMational Tips for Relationships:

Touch: Hug somebody every day—World-renowned family therapist, Virginia Satir, is quoted as saying "We need 4 hugs a day for survival. We need 8 hugs a day for maintenance. We need 12 hugs a day for growth."[155]

Shake hands and smile when greeting someone

Hold a friend's hand while you take time to talk with them

Have a massage or a manicure

Pet or hold a dog, cat, or bird

---

[152] *Creation Health: God's 8 Principles for living Life to the Fullest*, ed. Robyn Edgerton (Florida Hospital Mission Development, 2012), p. 165.
[153] Ibid.
[154] Ibid.
[155] Christine Comaford, Are You Getting Enough Hugs? Forbes, https://1ref.us/1rw.

Friendship: Be a friend and be friendly—look for the best in people and enthusiastically praise and encourage them for something good that they have accomplished. Put the "Golden Rule" into practice. "The heartfelt counsel of a friend is as sweet as perfume and incense" (Prov. 27:9, NLT).

> *Be a friend and be friendly—look for the best in people and enthusiastically praise and encourage them for something good that they have accomplished.*

Forgiveness: Think of someone who has wronged you and ask God to help you to forgive them. Continue to pray about them and yourself until you are able to truly let go of all animosity and forgive them. If possible, let them know that you have forgiven them. Enjoy the freedom that truly forgiving someone brings to your life!

Service to Others: Some time ago, I came across a quote which has given me excellent direction when it comes to service: "Don't ask yourself what the world needs. Ask yourself what makes you come alive, and go do that, because what the world needs is people who have come alive."[156]

Spend time volunteering in something that you are passionate about, and you have created a win-win situation!

---

[156] Howard Thurman, *The Living Wisdom of Howard Thurman: A Visionary for Our Time* (Sounds True Publishing, 2010).

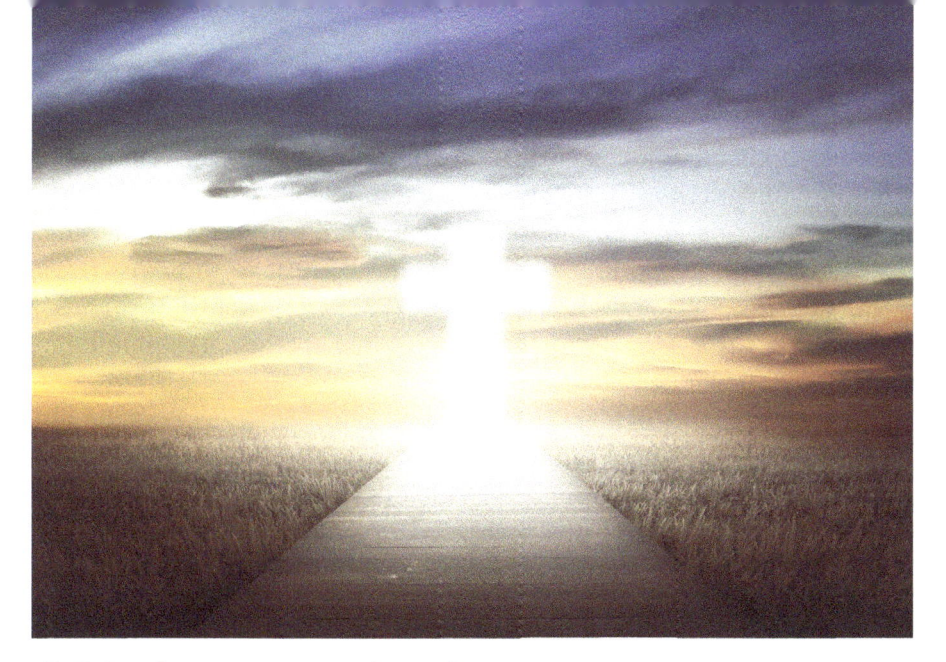

M is for ... Motivation

Our last letter in TRANSFORMing our health and our lives is M for Motivation. More than anything else that keeps that light burning brightly in our hearts is what is referred to as our purpose in life. What did God have in mind for you when you were created and grew up into the human family?

This is a question that burns in the hearts of many as they seek to find their way in this world. Some find it very early on, others find it after some time, and, sadly, there are many who never find it. It is my hope and prayer that, if you are one of those who has not yet found your way, that this chapter and this book may be of help to you in this most important part of your journey.

There is sufficient evidence to support the fact that being motivated with a purpose, a goal, a vision is a powerful and most necessary part of being whole, complete, and fulfilled as a person. And, not surprisingly, this motivating, driving force is what carries people through the worst, most harrowing experiences. It also delivers them onto the other side better, stronger, more focused, and more equipped to handle anything else that comes their way!

Take, for example, Viktor Frankl, a psychiatrist from Vienna who miraculously, it would appear, survived the Auschwitz Nazi concentration camp in World War II. Frankl found that survivors like himself had something to live for—"a golden thread of hope." Living through the most abominable, impossible conditions and suffering the worst that humans can inflict upon other humans, these death-camp survivors rose above the nightmare of Auschwitz by identifying something to live for and then taking positive action in achieving that dream. This, he discovered, is what makes life worth living. Frankl would go on to chronicle his experience in these death camps in his bestselling book, *Man's Search for Meaning*.[157] His book was to earn the distinction of being one of "the ten most influential books in the United States."[158]

"It is a peculiarity of man," wrote Frankl in his bestseller, "that he can only live by looking to the future …. And this is his salvation in the most difficult moments of his existence."[159]

I think of my friend's ninety-three-year-old mother-in-law who has books delivered to her to read each week and is active every day knitting hats and booties for premature babies at the hospital. This is what she lives for, and it keeps her mind and body active and alive. When my friend said that they might have to downsize from their house where she lives with them to an apartment, her response was, "OK, not a problem. I'll just get a condo and manage on my own!"

In his groundbreaking book, *The Blue Zones*, author Dan Buettner provides a list of nine lessons covering the lifestyles of the longest-living people groups on earth. The first lesson on that list is moderate, regular physical activity, and second is purpose.[160]

So, what is it that motivates you? What do you enjoy? What are you passionate about? One of the saddest things that I have observed in my life is talking to people who work at jobs they hate. These people are unfulfilled and life to them is just drudgery. We all know of those who retire and within a few months to a year, they are dead!

Motivation through Goal Setting

I am a huge believer in goal setting. According to a study done by David Kohl, professor emeritus at Virginia Tech, 80 percent of Americans report that they don't have goals. Some 16 percent say they do have goals, but they don't write them down. Less than 4 percent take the time to write down their goals, and less than 1 percent review them regularly. This small percentage of Americans who write down their goals and review them regularly, earn nine times more over the course of their lifetimes than those

---

157 Viktor Frankl, *Man's Search for Meaning* (Boston, MA: Beacon Press Publishing Company, 1963).
158 Esther Fein, "Book Notes," *New York Times*, https://1ref.us/1rx (accessed November 1, 2021).
159 Viktor Frankl, *Man's Search for Meaning* (Boston, MA: Beacon Press Publishing Company, 1963), pp. 115–116, 126.
160 Dan Buettner, *The Blue Zones*, 2nd ed. (National Geographic Books).

who don't set goals. This study alone should motivate you to write down your goals.[161]

How can the setting of goals be tailored to meet the Christian's need? Or does it need to be? What is the priority in the Christian experience? Do temporal needs supersede eternal realities? Answers to these questions should be given prayerful consideration when setting goals. God invites us to call upon Him for answers. *"'Call to Me and I will answer you, and show you great and mighty things, which you do not know'"* (Jer. 33:3).

Each January first, I take some time to prayerfully write out (it is important to actually handwrite, not type these out on your computer) my goals in all the important areas of my life for the coming year. These typically are (in no particular order of importance) personal; marriage and family goals; business and professional career; financial and investment goals; recreation. You can add others as you see fit.

Then in these categories, I break them up into subcategories such as in personal, I have my spiritual goals, fitness and athletic, health, personal and interpersonal growth, and hobbies. You can do the same for all categories. I find it makes it easier to compartmentalize into these subcategories so that you cover a broader range, and it keeps you working on all these different levels to grow as a person and most of all to keep motivated in a somewhat balanced way. This most certainly helps to give your life purpose.

If you took the time to do the Balance Wheel of Life near the beginning of this book, that is a good sign that you are indeed interested in where you are going in life and that you will probably take this seriously enough to take action. For those of you who didn't, my prayer is that reading this chapter will convince you that this is a vital part of growing and succeeding in life, and investing some time in this area will pay off in spades.

There is no actual wrong way to organize your goals—the main thing is to get them down on paper. Mark Victor Hansen used to always say, "Don't think it, ink it!"[162] I know seasoned goal setters who write out ten-year plans, five-year plans, three-year, and one-year plans and then break down the one year into quarters, monthly, weekly, and daily goals. Others just write down a handful of goals and focus on them. People are wired differently and so they will goal-set differently.

I have mentioned a few things about my personal approach to goal setting and we've looked at a comment Mark Victor Hansen has made

---

161 Jack Canfield and Janet Switzer, *The Success Principles: How to Get from Where You Are to Where You Want to Be* (New York, NY: HarperCollins Publishers, 2015), pp. 77–78.
162 Mark Victor Hansen, Quotetab, https://1ref.us/1ry (accessed October 28, 2021).

about this subject. Let us now compare what the Bible teaches regarding planning for the future/goal setting.

The biblical model of goal setting or planning includes asking of God to provide what we need for that day: *"Give us this day our daily bread"* (Matt. 6:11, KJV).

"So do not worry about tomorrow; for tomorrow will worry about itself. Each day has enough trouble of its own" (Matt. 6:34, AMP).

Similarly, James the brother of Jesus, reminds us: *"Now listen, you who say, "Today or tomorrow we will go to this or that city, spend a year there, carry on business and make money." Why, you do not even know what will happen tomorrow. What is your life? You are a mist that appears for a little while and then vanishes. Instead, you ought to say, "If it is the Lord's will, we will live and do this or that"* (James 4:13–15, NIV).

As evidenced by these verses, there is a marked contrast between secular and spiritual models of goal setting. I encourage a balanced approach, allowing God to give the correct expectation. Understanding this, we will not become discouraged if or when there is a need to adjust our goals.

It is important that you find your own groove and not feel overwhelmed in your goal setting. For some, having multiple goals works well, while for others, having just one or a few is plenty.

I encourage you to stretch yourself by dreaming as big as you can and set a breakthrough goal or what Jack Canfield calls a Big, Hairy, Audacious Goal or BHAG.[163] Unlike most other goals, where you chip away at them each day, the BHAG is going to take a huge amount of focus, time, and effort and will likely need the greater part of your daily attention. My BHAG for this year was to write and publish this very book you are reading and it has indeed taken the better part of my spare time.

Set SMART Goals

There is, however, a right and a wrong way to phrase your goals. When I write out my goals, I like to use the SMART acronym. The goal needs to be Specific, Measurable, Attainable, Relevant, and Timely.

Here is an example of what I mean by a SMART goal. Suppose you want to lose weight. You need to decide how much weight. Let's say you weigh 165 pounds, and you want to lose twenty-five pounds. Here is how a SMART goal should be worded: "I will weigh 140 pounds on or before _____ (put in a realistic date). This is specific and measurable. Twenty-five pounds should be attainable; it is relevant to your needs and desires,

---

[163] Facebook, December 14, 2011, https://1ref.us/1rz (accessed October 28, 2021).

and it has a completion date. Notice the use of "I will," not "I would like to," in order to add certainty to the accomplishment of the goal.

Write out as much detail as possible. For example, if your family is growing out of that starter home, picture in your mind the new home that you would like to purchase in vivid detail—its location, how it looks, the landscaping, the rooms, everything you can conjure up in your mind. Then write it all down in detail so that your subconscious mind can faithfully record what it is and make you more acutely aware of opportunities that will lead you step-by-step to your goal. Cutting out a picture of a home that somewhat resembles what you have in mind is a powerful tool to give the goal more credibility to your belief.

As a Christian, I believe my goals should not be presumptuous or selfish or unduly materialistic. I believe that I want to be praying for the Lord's guidance in the goals I set so that they would be within the Lord's will and purpose for me in my life. In addition, I want my goals to fully utilize all the gifts, talents, and skills that I have been blessed with. Then, each day, it is important to review each goal, being reminded that they are placed before the One who is able to bring it to fruition, praying over them upon rising and upon retiring. That way, you are assured that your goals remain upon the altar of faith to be pursued or given up as God's providence unfolds.

Use God's Promises to Overcome Negative Self-Talk

Every waking moment of every day, our minds are constantly at work processing a myriad of things at once. One of those functions is what is called *self-talk*, which are the words or pictures that our mind is repeating over and over. For most of us, self-talk can be negative and pessimistic at times and counterproductive to a healthy self-image.

Claiming God's promises is a wonderful way to refute negative self-talk and further reinforce in your mind that your goals are bound up in Christ. Claiming God's promises establishes truth that God already sees His goal for you in its completed state.

For example, if your negative self-talk is constantly babbling to you that you are overweight and unattractive at 150 pounds, claim confidently, "I am enjoying the assurance of being slim and trim at 125 pounds because … *"I can do all things through Christ who strengthens me"* (Phil. 4:13).

If your self-talk is nattering at you about a certain health problem or symptom you are experiencing, you can claim the promise of Psalm 103:2–3: *"Bless the LORD, O my soul, and forget not all His benefits: who forgives all your iniquities, who heals all your diseases.*" I am 100 percent healthy in Him.

For undesirable thoughts that enter your mind, you can say "It is written," claiming the promise in the Bible that refutes the enemies lies about that subject. Even better is to be proactive by replacing that negative thought or statement with a positive one. For example, if your self-talk is saying that your forgetfulness is worsening every day, replace it with a promise such as *"For God has not given us a spirit of fear, but of power and of love and of a sound mind"* (2 Tim. 1:7), or *"I will praise You, for I am fearfully and wonderfully made"* (Ps. 139:14). Apply this principle of claiming God's promises to all negative thoughts and see how you improve rather than worsen.

> *For undesirable thoughts that enter your mind, you can say "It is written," claiming the promise in the Bible that refutes the enemies lies about that subject. Even better is to be proactive by replacing that negative thought or statement with a positive one.*

In instances where you have attempted to say or do something and it just didn't go right, instead of beating yourself up, simply say to yourself, "Next time, I ...." or "That's not like me ...." Ask yourself, "What is the lesson learned here? How can I grow in and through this?"

How to Claim God's Promises Effectively and Intelligently

Be sure to use the present tense and be specific. Claim God's promise that addresses a current experience. For example, "Lord I am writing my_____ exam today. I have prepared for it according to the best of my ability and, therefore, I claim your wisdom as promised in 1 Corinthians 1:30, BSB, for any shortfall that may arise. *"It is because of Him that you are in Christ Jesus, who has become for us wisdom from God: our righteousness, holiness and redemption."*

State it in the positive. Claim what you want, not what you don't want. The Scriptures teach us to, *"Ask and it will be given to you; seek and you will find; knock and the door will be opened to you. For everyone who asks receives; the one who seeks finds; and to the one who knocks, the door will be opened"* (Matt. 7:7–8, NIV).

How to Create Effective Affirmations

Affirmations are positive statements that can help you to challenge and overcome self-sabotaging and negative thoughts. When you repeat them often, and believe in them, you can start to make positive changes. For your affirmations to be effective, certain guidelines are very useful. The following is borrowed largely from Jack Canfield's classic book, *The Success Principles*.[164]

Start with the words "**I am**."

Use the **present tense**.

State it in the **positive**. Affirm **what you want,** not what you don't want.

Keep it **brief**.

Make it **specific**.
Wrong: I am enjoying my new clothes.
Right: I am enjoying my new navy pinstripe suit.

Include an **action word** ending with *-ing*.
Wrong: I express myself openly and honestly.
*Right: I am confidently **expressing** myself openly and honestly.*

Include at least **one dynamic emotion or feeling word.** Include the emotional state you would be feeling if you had already achieved the goal. Some commonly used words are *enjoying, joyfully, happily, celebrating, proudly, calmly, peacefully, delighted, enthusiastic, lovingly, secure, serenely, and triumphant.*

Make affirmations **for yourself, not others**.
Wrong: I am watching Johnny clean up his room.
Right: I am effectively communicating my needs and desires to Johnny.

Add: *"If it is according to Your will, Lord"* or *"Or something better according to Your will, O Lord"* when it is appropriate. When you are affirming a specific situation, such as getting a new job, opportunity, vacation, material object (e.g., house, car, boat), or relationship (husband, wife, child), always add the words: *"If it is according to Your will, Lord"* or *"Or something better according to Your will, O Lord."* As Christians, we want our goals and affirmations to be in perfect harmony with what the Lord wants and knows is best for us.

---
[164] Ibid pp. 101–105.

E.g., I am happily employed working for the _____ Marketing Agency or something better according to Your will, O Lord.

The Lord may have something in mind for us that is *better* or *better suited for us and what He wants us to do*. For the believer, God always gives us what we ask for or something better, according to His will. Isn't that a wonderful promise? If what we have asked for is not granted, we must remember that the Lord knows what is and isn't good for us or He may grant this at some later time.

So now you have your guidelines for making affirmations. Again, like your goals, they should be written out in detail and placed on the altar of faith, trusting the One who is able to bring them into reality.

Trusting God's will as being paramount and that you have given Him permission to remain there to guide you and create opportunity, will most certainly drive away negative self-talk. Once you are settled in this, you will experience yourself being aligned with Christ, your ignorance connected to His wisdom, your weakness to His strength, your fear to His courage. The mind of Christ is a powerful cohesion of thought, action, and creation, bringing about fulfillment of the statements that you have asked for and claimed. In His authority, things have been set in motion. It is indeed amazing when you harness the power of the mind of Christ rather than the typical human negative default.

Revolutionize Your Prayer Life

As Christians, we know that prayer is vitally important in our spiritual experience for many reasons. For one thing, Jesus, who is our example, prayed often. The Bible reveals that sometimes Jesus would spend an entire night in prayer: *"And it came to pass in those days, that he went out into a mountain to pray, and continued all night in prayer to God"* (Luke 6:12, KJV). If Jesus felt the need to pray as much as He did, it seems that we, in our sinful human condition, might consider that prayer might be of even *more* importance to us.

Jesus communed with His Father in prayer for all things. None of what He did was independent of the Father. *"I can of mine own self do nothing: as I hear, I judge: and my judgment is just; because I seek not mine own will, but the will of the Father which hath sent me"* (John 5:30, KJV). As mentioned above, as a follower of Jesus, this is something else we can implement in our own prayer life. In practically all of my prayers, I preface or conclude them with the words of Jesus: *"[N]ot my will, but thine, be done"* (Luke 22:42, KJV).

Not only that, but after His resurrection, Jesus gave His disciples (and all of us just for the asking) the promised gift of the Holy Spirit: *"Then He breathed on them, and said, 'Receive the Holy Spirit'"* (John 20:22, NLT).

Remember, it is the Holy Spirit that makes intercession. The Spirit also helps our infirmities because we know not what we should pray for, but the Spirit itself makes intercession for us with groanings which cannot be expressed in words (Rom. 8:26, paraphrase). *"Now He who searches the hearts knows what the mind of the Spirit is, because He makes intercession for the saints [i.e., believers] according to the will of God"* (Rom. 8:27).

Prayer is the outpouring of the heart to our heavenly Father, and, as mentioned above, when we know not how to pray, the Holy Spirit makes intercession for us. Jesus gave a model of prayer when asked by His disciples how to pray. That prayer can be found in Matthew 6:9–13, often called "the Lord's Prayer."

Understanding the power of prayer motivates us to *pray for others* as well as for ourselves. As these prayers of intercession go up, it can be the most rewarding experience in our spiritual lives as we literally see God intervening and interceding in the lives and experience of those for whom we are praying.

Prayers to God take on many forms including supplications, which is defined as asking or begging for something earnestly or humbly. The prayers of supplication and petition could be considered biblical affirmations.

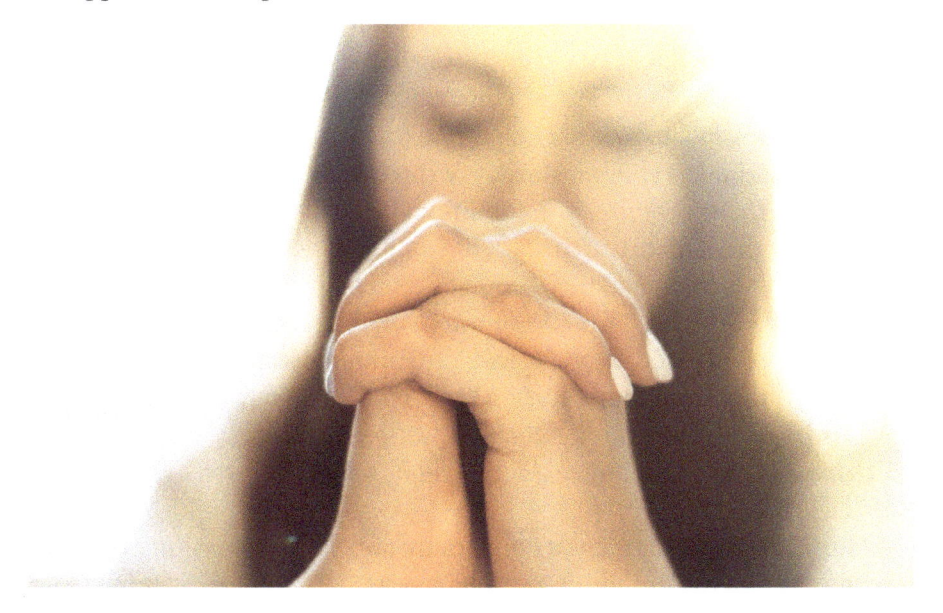

I like to use a simple formula called the **ABCs of prayer**. **'A' means Ask** (*"Ask and it will be given to you; seek and you will find; knock and the door will be opened to you"* (Matt. 7:7, NIV)). **'B' means Believe** that the LORD will grant your request, and **'C' means to Claim** it. Then couple this with a Bible promise (of which there are 5,467 found in Scripture[165]) to add tremendous power to your prayers.

What we typically do is, if we have a problem, like a bad temper, we pray to ask God to help us deal with it or get rid of it. We go on and on about how troublesome it is to us. However, the Lord is not interested in being part of the problem, but rather, He wants to be part of the solution. So how could we approach it then with the solution in mind? The opposite of being bad-tempered is being peaceful in our thoughts, words, and actions, so we would search for a Bible promise that would have to do with our being peaceful.

Isaiah chapter 26 and verse 3 says (NLT), "You will keep in perfect peace all who trust in you, all whose thoughts are fixed on you!" So, you would pray "Lord, I ASK for You to give me a peaceful mind. Lord, I BELIEVE You will give me peace in my thoughts, words, and actions, and (CLAIM it) I am receiving Your peace, O Lord, as You promised in Isaiah 26:3."

We can apply this to any prayer request, as long as we keep in mind two things: First, we must understand that faith is a gift from God. "For by grace are ye saved through faith; and that [faith] not of yourselves: it is the gift of God" (Eph. 2:8, KJV). Only through exercise of this faith can God bring about the things we ask of Him. Hebrews 11:6 states: "But without faith it is impossible to please Him, for he who comes to God must believe that He is, and that He is a rewarder of those who diligently seek Him."

Second, these promises are conditional in that it is only IN CHRIST that we are privileged to receive God's abundance. Christ's obedience that secured God's abundance becomes ours by faith. *"All praise to God, the Father of our Lord Jesus Christ, who has blessed us with every spiritual blessing in the heavenly realms because we are united with Christ"* (Eph. 1:3, NLT). It is, therefore, our choice whether we choose to accept or reject the Lord and His promises. *"But seek ye first the kingdom of God, and **his righteousness**; and all these things shall be **added** unto you"* (Matt. 6:33, KJV).

Our heavenly Father knows our frailty and He is always interested in hearing the honest outpouring of our hearts. His comfort is refreshing,

---

[165] "5467 promises, divine," Bible Gateway, https://1ref.us/1s0 (accessed November 1, 2021).

"For I know the plans I have for you, declares the LORD, plans to prosper you and not to harm you, to give you a future and a hope" (Jer. 29:11, BSB). He loves us more than words can describe and wants to answer our prayers as we humbly come to Him, believing that He will answer our prayers according to His will.

With tender pity, He invites us to come and reason with Him. Isaiah 1:18 (KJV) says, *"Come now, and let us reason together, saith the LORD: though your sins be as scarlet, they shall be as white as snow; though they be red like crimson, they shall be as wool."*

God's promises are irrevocable, and He is absolutely trustworthy. He is unchanging and is faithful in keeping *all* His promises. Since the Lord Jesus is committed, willing, and eager to bless us (see 2 Cor. 9:8–10) and because the gift is in the promise, God is faithful to answer our prayer *according to His will and in His own time.*

Other prayer requests you might consider asking for are forgiveness, wisdom, salvation, and much, much more.

- "I'm claiming you, Jesus, as my forgiveness as promised in 1 John 1:9." ("If we confess our sins, He is faithful and just to forgive us *our* sins and to cleanse us from all unrighteousness.")
- "I'm claiming you, Jesus, as my wisdom as promised in James 1:5." ("If any of you lacks wisdom, you should ask God, who gives generously to all without finding fault, and it will be given to you.")
- "I'm claiming you, Jesus, as my salvation as promised in Ephesians 2:8–9." ("For by grace you have been saved through faith, and that not of yourselves; *it is* the gift of God, not of works, lest anyone should boast.")
- "I'm claiming you, Jesus, to be the Savior of my family as promised in Psalm 2 verse 8." ("Ask of me, and I shall give thee the heathen for thine inheritance, and the uttermost parts of the earth for thy possession" (KJV).)

The Nine Types of Motivation[166]

There are two main types of motivation and seven more minor forms.

1. Intrinsic Motivation—This is a type of motivation where a person is driven by internal desires. For example, if Janet wants to lose weight to feel healthier and to be happier with her appearance,

---

166 Buckley, D. "9 Types of Motivation That Make It Possible to Reach Your Dreams," https://1ref.us/1s1 (accessed October 28, 2021).

then this is an intrinsic type of motivation because Janet's desire to change comes from within.

2. Extrinsic Motivation—Opposite to intrinsic, extrinsic motivation comes from external influences and desires. In this case, Janet's husband has been hinting that perhaps if she trimmed off some of that excess weight, she might be more attractive to him.

3. Reward-Based or Incentive Motivation—This and the other more minor forms of motivation fall into either intrinsic or extrinsic motivation. A reward incentivizes one to complete a task or project or reach a sales target, for example, because they know that there is something they will receive on completion of that task. The bigger the reward, the greater the motivation.

4. Fear-Based Motivation—This type is not based on the negative word "fear" so much as it is based on the "fear of failure." Seasoned goal-setters know that accountability is a powerful motivator. Not wanting to let someone down or look less than ideal to those you hold in high esteem can move a person to follow through on achieving that goal.

5. Achievement-Based Motivation—There are those who like to take on something just for the sake of achievement. They may want to improve professionally, so they take a course even though this may or may not enhance their position or improve their income. For some, this just keeps them active and constantly learning and growing.

6. Power-Based Motivation—This seems to bring to mind someone who is power-hungry and only cares for his or her self-advancement as an end to gain more power, control, and/or money. This is viewed by most people as an undesirable form of motivation—which it is. However, for the person who has in him or herself a burning desire to effect change in the world around them, gaining positions of power or influence can help bring this into reality. This type of power Christ received from the Father to heal our suffering planet. *"And Jesus came and spake unto them, saying, All power is given unto me in heaven and in earth"* (Matt. 28:18, KJV). *"As thou hast given him power over all flesh, that he should give eternal life to as many as thou hast given him"* (John 17:2, KJV).

7. Affiliation Motivation—Who is it that motivates you? Who inspires you? Is there someone you look up to who motivates you

to do better, work harder, to accomplish great things? Affiliation motivation is the motivation someone has to connect with another whom they deem to be at a higher level or position to achieve their goals. It is even more satisfying when that person compliments the work they have done or the achievement they have accomplished. The apostle Paul says that the love of Christ motivates His disciples. *"For the love of Christ compels us, because we judge thus: that if One died for all, then all died; and He died for all, that those who live should live no longer for themselves, but for Him who died for them and rose again"* (2 Cor. 5:14–15).

8. Competence Motivation—If you have ever thought you wanted to improve at something such as an aspect of your job or improve at a sport or learn a musical instrument, competence motivation is what you will need to succeed here. Oftentimes, an obstacle or a sticky issue will motivate you to search out an answer to resolve the problem.

9. Attitude Motivation—If you are not happy with your attitude, outlook, or beliefs and this is holding you back in life, some attitude motivation will be needed to recover and move forward properly. If you intensely desire to change the way that you see things around you or the way you see yourself, setting goals associated with self-awareness and self-change will be met with attitude motivation.[167]

Are You a Motivator?

In a way, we are all motivators, either at home or at work—whether we're persuading a friend to lose weight or giving a pep talk to our kids or in baseball trying to help a batter out of a slump, we're motivators.[168]

There are many people who find fulfillment in helping others, inspiring, encouraging, coaching, and motivating people to success in their lives. Turning your passion into a career is a great way to fulfill your purpose.

Extra TRANSFORMational Tips for Motivation:

1. Search your heart and ask the Lord to reveal to you your purpose or mission in life. King Solomon concluded that the epitome of motivation was for mankind to fulfill our role as ministers of

---
167 Ibid.,
168 Alan Loy McGinnis, *Bringing Out the Best in People* (Minneapolis, MN: Augsburg Publishing House, 1985), p. 14.

God. *"Let us hear the conclusion of the whole matter: Fear God, and keep his commandments: for this is the whole duty of man"* (Eccles. 12:13, KJV). Isaiah states it this way: *"You are my witnesses," says the LORD, "And My servant whom I have chosen, that you may know and believe Me and understand that I am He. Before Me there was no God formed, nor shall there be after Me"* (Isa. 43:10).

"Arise, shine, for your light has come, and the glory of the LORD has risen upon you. For behold, darkness shall cover the earth, and thick darkness the peoples; but the LORD will arise upon you, and his glory will be seen upon you. And nations shall come to your light, and kings to the brightness of your rising" (Isa. 60:1–3, ESV).

2. Many authors have written excellent books on motivation, inspiration, life purpose, personal discovery, and growth. These have been of practical value to me, and you may find they teach you new ways to keep your passion burning. Some suggestions are the *Chicken Soup for the Soul* series as well as books by John Maxwell, Jack Canfield, Stan Toler, Les Brown, Og Mandino, and many others. Attend a seminar at least once a year devoted to growing personally. For the greatest true motivation, however, we turn from lesser motivators to God. Understanding that our main purpose is to make God known to a world that does not know Him will bring joy and motivation, fulfillment in every aspect of our lives. We can submit to God and allow Him to develop us according to the ability He has blessed us with. Isn't that powerful motivation?

"The fear of the LORD is the beginning of wisdom, and knowledge of the Holy One is understanding" (Prov. 9:10, NIV).

3. The following quotes from one of my favorite authors will expand upon this thought found in Proverbs.

The world has had its great teachers, men of giant intellect and extensive research, men whose utterances have stimulated thought and opened to view vast fields of knowledge; and these men have been honored as guides and benefactors of their race; but there is One who stands higher than they. We can trace the line of the world's teachers as far back as human records extend; but the Light was before them. As the moon and the stars of our solar system shine by the reflected light of the sun, so, as far as their teaching is true, do the world's great thinkers reflect the rays of the Sun of Righteousness.

Every gleam of thought, every flash of the intellect, is from the Light of the world.[169]

True education means more than the pursual of a certain course of study. It means more than a preparation for the life that now is. It has to do with the whole being, and with the whole period of existence possible to man. It is the harmonious development of the physical, the mental, and the spiritual powers. It prepares the student for the joy of service in this world and for the higher joy of wider service in the world to come.[170]

In a knowledge of God all true knowledge and real development have their source. Wherever we turn, in the physical, the mental, or the spiritual realm; in whatever we behold, apart from the blight of sin, this knowledge is revealed. Whatever line of investigation we pursue, with a sincere purpose to arrive at truth, we are brought in touch with the unseen, mighty Intelligence that is working in and through all. The mind of man is brought into communion with the mind of God, the finite with the Infinite. The effect of such communion on body and mind and soul is beyond estimate.[171]

4. Read biographies and autobiographies of famous, successful people whose lives will inspire you and motivate you to greater things.

5. Many will feel they are losing their way due to the setbacks and discouragements with which life presents us. You must not only anticipate this, you must expect it. Pray earnestly that the Lord will give you strength and fortitude to withstand these challenges. Know that if you are attempting anything in the spiritual realm, the enemy, Satan, will do his best to take you down in whatever way he can. Remember that Jesus Christ is all-powerful and one with God, and He has already defeated the devil and his evil plans by dying for us at the cross. Claim His name and His promises constantly throughout your day. A good Scripture for victory is *"If God is for us, who can be against us?"* (Rom. 8:31). Never forget that anything of value in this life takes effort, determination, and persistence. Of course, in turning to the Lord for supplication, these values that Christ has gifted you with will be ever greater accomplished in Him. I speak from experience on that!

---

169 Ellen G. White, *Education* (Mountain View, CA: Pacific Press, 1903), pp. 13–14.
170 Ibid., p. 13.
171 Ibid., p. 14.

> Many whom God has qualified to do excellent work accomplish very little, because they attempt little. Thousands pass through life as if they had no definite object for which to live, no standard to reach. Such will obtain a reward proportionate to their works. Remember that you will never reach a higher standard than you yourself set …. Press with determination in the right direction, and circumstances will be your helpers, not your hindrances.[172] —Ellen G. White

Food for Thought: *"So utterly was Christ emptied of self that He made no plans for Himself. He accepted God's plans for Him, and day by day the Father unfolded His plans. So should we depend on God, that our lives may be the simple outworking of His will."*[173]

---

172 Ellen G. White, *Christ's Object Lessons* (Washington, DC: Review and Herald, 1900), pp. 331–332.
173 Ellen G. White, *The Desire of Ages* (Mountain View, CA: Pacific Press, 1898), p. 208.

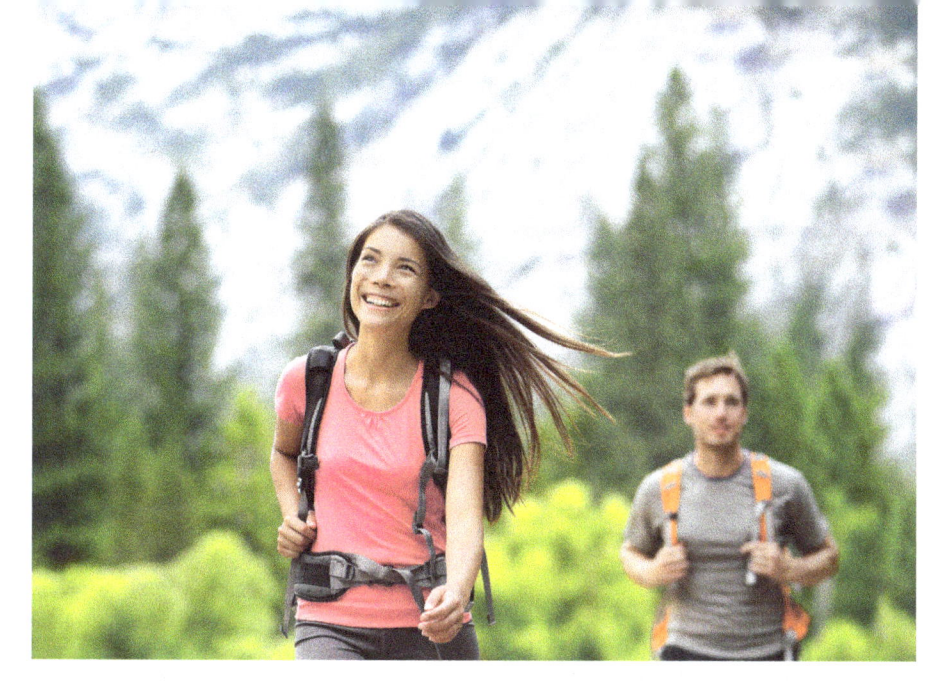

Conclusion

So, now you have the prescription to take your health and your life to the next level and beyond.

I promise you, that if you take these principles seriously, the Lord will richly bless you in ways that you cannot even fathom right now. I have incorporated, and am continuing to incorporate, these into my own life, and my gratitude for the richness that TRANSFORM has brought me can only be described as revolutionary.

It is my hope and wish that as you prayerfully institute even just one or part of one of these fundamentals into your life that you, too, will be blessed bountifully. Don't be discouraged if you fall off—just course correct and keep going. We are all on a journey—and it is the work of a lifetime.

I would like to finish off with something that has been very inspirational for me called "A Creed to Live By" by Nancye Sims. I believe it encapsulates a number of things I have discussed, especially the latter half of the book dealing with outlook, relationships, and motivation.

A Creed to Live By

Don't undermine your worth by comparing yourself with others.

It is because we are different that each of us is special.

Don't set your goals by what other people deem important.

Only you know what is best for you.

Don't take for granted the things closest to your heart.

Cling to them as you would your life,

for without them life is meaningless.

Don't let your life slip through your fingers

by living in the past or for the future

By living your life one day at a time,

you live all the days of your life.

Don't give up when you still have something to give.

Nothing is really over...until the moment you stop trying.

Don't be afraid to admit that you are less than perfect.

It is a fragile thread that binds us to each other.

Don't be afraid to encounter risks.

It is by taking chances that we learn how to be brave.

Don't shut love out of your life by saying it's impossible to find.

The quickest way to receive love is to give love;

the fastest way to lose love is to hold it too tightly;

and the best way to keep love is to give it wings.

Don't dismiss your dreams.

To be without dreams is to be without hope;

to be without hope is to be without purpose.

Don't run through life so fast

that you forget not only where you've been

but also where you're going.

Life is not a race, but a journey **to be savoured**

each step of the way.

Just remember ... don't stop going and don't stop growing. Consecrate each day of your life to the Lord, asking that in Him, you can make this day and every day a Masterpiece.

Dr. David Sloan, M.H., PhD., DNM, RNT.

For contact information, enter this link in your web browser: https://1ref.us/r9457062

Bibliography

"10 Surprising Health Benefits of Walking Barefoot." Power of Positivity. https://1ref.us/1qn.

"5467 promises, divine." Bible Gateway. https://1ref.us/1s0.

"Agriculture: cause and victim of water pollution, but change is possible." Food and Agriculture Organization of the United Nations. https://1ref.us/1r2.

Allen, Karen M., Jim Blascovich, Joe Tomaka, and Robert M. Kelsey. "Presence of human friends and pet dogs as moderators of autonomic responses to stress in women." *Journal of Personality and Social Psychology*. Vol. 61, Issue 4 (1991).

American Academy of Sleep Medicine. "Obstructive Sleep Apnea." https://1ref.us/1qj.

American Osteopathic Association. "Low magnesium levels make vitamin D ineffective: Up to 50 percent of US population is magnesium deficient." ScienceDaily. https://1ref.us/1ri.

Arnarson, Atli. "7 Signs and Symptoms of Magnesium Deficiency." https://1ref.us/1rk.

Ayas, N. "A Prospective Study of Self-Reported Sleep Duration and Incident Type 2 Diabetes in Women." *Diabetes Care* 26 (2003).

Ayas, Najib et al. "A Prospective Study of Sleep Duration and Coronary Heart Disease in Women." *Journal Archives of Internal Medicine* 163 (2003).

"10 benefits of walking with barefoot." https://1ref.us/1qp.

Beck, Melinda. "Selenium as an antiviral agent." Springer Link. https://1ref.us/1rh.

Beers, Mark H., and Robert Berkow. *The Merck Manual of Geriatrics.* Whitehouse Station, NJ: Merck Research Laboratories, 2009.

Benson, Herbert, and Marg Stark. *Timeless Healing: The Power and Biology of Belief.* New York, NY: Fireside (Scribner), 1997.

Biello, David. "Laughter Proves Good Medicine for Heart." *Scientific American*. https://1ref.us/1rq.

Boot, Walter R., and Arthur F. Kramer. "The Brain-Games Conundrum: Does Cognitive Training Really Sharpen the Mind?" NCBI. https://1ref.us/1qt.

Buettner, Dan. *The Blue Zones.* 2nd ed. National Geographic Books, 2012.

Canfield, Jack, and Janet Switzer. *The Success Principles: How to Get from Where You Are to Where You Want to Be*. New York, NY: HarperCollins Publishers, 2015.

Carrington, Damian, and George Arnett. "Clear Differences between organic and non-organic food, study finds." *The Guardian*. https://1ref.us/1r4.

Chef AJ. "Can Heart Disease be Reversed? | Interview with Dr. Hans Diehl." https://1ref.us/1r0.

Chesworth, Ward, Felipe Macias-Vasquez, David Acquaye, and Edmond Thompson. "Agriculture Alchemy: Stones into Bread." *Episodes - Journal of International Geoscience* 1983.

Chevalier, Gaetan, Stephen T. Sinatra, and Pawel Sokal. "Earthing: Health Implications of Reconnecting the Human Body to the Earth's Surface Electrons." *Journal of Environmental and Public Health* (2012).

Chowdhury, Madhuleena R. "The Neuroscience of Gratitude and How It Affects Anxiety and Grief." Positive Psychology. https://1ref.us/1qb.

Colburn, Don. "Norman Cousins, Still Laughing." *The Washington Post*, October 21, 1986.

Comaford, Christine. "Are You Getting Enough Hugs?" *Forbes*. https://1ref.us/1rw.

Cousins, Norman. *Anatomy of An Illness as Perceived by the Patient: Reflections on Healing and Regeneration.* New York, NY: Norton Publishing, 1979.

Cousins, Norman. *Head First: The Biology of Hope.* New York, NY: E.P. Dutton, 1989.

Creation Health: God's 8 Principles for living Life to the Fullest. Edited by Robyn Edgerton. Florida Hospital Mission Development, 2012.

Cronkleton, Emily. "Why Being Flexible Is Great for Your Health." healthline. https://1ref.us/1qr.

Dashti, Hussein M., et al. "Long-term effects of a ketogenic diet in obese patients." *Experimental and Clinical Cardiology* 9, (2004).

Dossey, Larry, *Meaning and Medicine: Lessons from a Doctor's Tales of Breakthrough and Healing.* New York, NY: Bantam Books, 1991.

Ducharme, Jamie. "5 Places Where People Live the Longest and Healthiest Lives." February 15, 2018, https://1ref.us/1qk.

Ducharme, Jamie. "U.S. Suicide Rates Are the Highest They've Been Since World War II." *TIME*. https://1ref.us/1qa.

El-Hamd, Mohammed Abu and Soha Aboeldahab. "Cell phone and male infertility: An update," *Journal of Nephrology and Andrology*. https://1ref.us/1qg.

Ellis, Ralph. "Pandemic Screen Time: Will Blue Light Glasses Help?" WebMD. https://1ref.us/1qi.

Fein, Esther. "Book Notes." *New York Times*. https://1ref.us/1rx.

Fielding, Sarah. "New Study Shows 91 Percent of Fears Don't Come True." BestLife. https://1ref.us/1s2.

Ford, Henry. "Whether you think you can, or you think you can't—you're right." *Harrisburg Telegraph:* November 1947.

Frankl, Viktor. *Man's Search for Meaning.* Boston, MA: Beacon Press Publishing Company, 1963.

Frazier, Linda M. "Reproductive disorders associated with pesticide exposure." *J Agromedicine*, no. 12 (2007), https://1ref.us/1r1.

Ghaly, Maurice, and Dale Teplitz. "The biologic effects of grounding the human body during sleep as measured by cortisol levels and subjective reporting of sleep, pain and stress." *Journal of Alternative and Complementary Medicine* 10 (2004).

"Good news if you buy organic food—it's getting cheaper." *Associated Press*, January 24, 2019.

Hartz-Seeley, Deborah S. "Chronic stress is linked to the six leading causes of death." Miami Hauser, Annie. "Vegetarians Live Longer, Study Finds." Wellness. https://1ref.us/1qw.

Hartz-Seeley, Deborah. "Chronic Stress Is Linked to the Six Leading Causes of Death." *Miami Herald*, March 21, 2014. https://1ref.us/1qe.

Harvard Health Letter. "Blue Light Has a Dark Side." Harvard Health Publishing. https://1ref.us/1s3.

Hill, Napoleon. *Think and Grow Rich.* New York, NY: Fawcett Books, 1987.

Holtz, Lou. goodreads. https://1ref.us/1rn.

"Hormone Vitamin D." Hormone Health Network. https://1ref.us/1rd.

Howell, Andrew, Jesse C. Jährig, and Russell A. Powell. "Sleep quality, sleep propensity and academic performance." *Perceptual & Motor Skills* (October 2004).

"How Much Sugar Do You Eat? You May Be Surprised!" https://1ref.us/1r6.

Idler, Ellen L., and Stanislav Karl. "Health perceptions and survival: do global evaluations of health status really predict mortality?" *Journal of Gerontology* 46 (1991).

Iodine, Selenium Deficiency and Kashin-Beck Disease. Edited by Victor R. Preedy, Gerard N. Burrow, and Ronald Watson. Elsevier Inc, 2009, Comprehensive Handbook of Iodine.

International Journal of Sport Science. "New Study: Rebounding Burns Fat And Improves Cardio Better Than Running." bellicon. https://1ref.us/1qu.

Kargar, Saeed, Seyed Mostafa Shiryazdi, and Mahdieh Kamali. "Urinary Iodine Concentrations in Cancer Patients." *Asian Pacific Journal of Cancer Prevention* 18 (2017).

Keltner, Dacher. "Hands On Research: The Science of Touch." *Greater Good Magazine.* https://1ref.us/1rt.

Koenig, H.G., M. McCullough, and D.B. Larson. *Handbook of religion and health: a century of research reviewed.* New York, NY: Oxford University Press, 2001.

Koenig, H.G. "Religion, Spirituality and Health: The Research and Clinical Implications." *ISRN Psychiatry* (2012).

Kubala, Jillian. "7 Science-Based Health Benefits of Selenium." healthline. https://1ref.us/1rg.

Kuburi, Julia. "9 Surprising Health Benefits of Walking Barefoot." Medium. https://1ref.us/1qq.

Levi, F., and F. Halberg. "Circaseptan (about-7-day) bioperiodicity—spontaneous and reactive—and the search for pacemakers." *Ric Clin Lab* 12 (1982).

Levin, J. *God, Faith and Health: Exploring the Spirituality-Healing Connection.* New York, NY: John Wiley and Sons, Inc., 2001.

Levin, J., and C. Ellison. "Modeling Religious Effects on Health and Psychological Well-Being: A replicated Secondary Data Analysis of Seven Study Samples." Unpublished research quoted in J. Levin, *God, Faith and Health*.

Levin, J., L. Chatters, et al. "Religious Effects on Health Status and Life Satisfaction Among Black Americans." *Journal of Gerontology: Social Sciences* 50B (1995).

Litovitz, T. A. "Bioeffects induced by exposure to microwaves are mitigated by superposition of ELF noise." *Bioelectromagnetics* 18, no. 6 (1997).

Litovitz, T. A., et al. "Superimposing spatially coherent electromagnetic noise inhibits field-induced abnormalities in developing chick embryos." *Bioeletromagnetics* 15 (1994).

"Magnesium in diet." MedlinePlus. https://1ref.us/1rj.

Martin, Rod A. "Do Children Laugh Much More Often than Adults Do?" Association for Applied and Therapeutic Humor. https://1ref.us/1rr.

Maruta, Toshihiko, Robert C. Colligan, Michael Malinchoc, and Kenneth P. Offord. "Optimists versus Pessimists: Survival Rate Among Patients over a 30-Year Period." *Mayo Clinic Proceedings* 75 (2000).

Mastroianni, Brian. "Binge-Watching TV May Be Dulling Your Brain." healthline. https://1ref.us/1qs.

McCullough, M. E., R. A. Emmons, and J. Tsang. "The Grateful Disposition: A Conceptual and Empirical Topography." *Journal of Personality and Social Psychology* 82 (2002).

McFarland, K. *The Lucifer Files.* Boise, ID: Pacific Press Publishing Association, 1988.

"Mental Imagery." Physiopedia. https://1ref.us/1rp.

McGinnis, Alan Loy. *Bringing Out the Best in People.* Minneapolis, MN: Augsburg Publishing House, 1985.

Miller, Aaron. "'In God We Trust' a motto or more?" The Clarion. https://1ref.us/1qd.

Moore, Thomas J. *Prescription for Disaster.* New York, NY: Simon and Schuster: Rockefeller Center, 1998.

Morin, Monte, "Organic foods are more nutritious according to review of 343 studies." *Los Angeles Times.* https://1ref.us/1r3.

Musick, M. "Religion and Subjective Health Among Black and White Elders." *Journal of Health and Social Behaviour* 37 (1996).

Nelson, Miriam. *Strong Women Stay Young.* New York, NY: Bantam Books, 1997.

"New Survey Reveals More than Half of Americans are Living with Gastrointestinal Symptoms and Not Seeking Care from a Doctor." Abbvie. https://1ref.us/1qy.

News Company. "5 Benefits of Lean Muscle Mass Besides a Good Physique." https://1ref.us/1r9.

New World Encyclopedia. "Nicaragua." https://1ref.us/1qc.

Null, G., Feldman M., Rasio D., and Dean C. *Death By Medicine.* Revised ed. Mount Jackson, VA: Prakitos Books, 2011.

Ober, Clinton, Stephen T. Sinatra, and Martin Zucker. "Earthing: The Most Important Health Discovery Ever?" *Basic Health Publications* (2010).

Obomsawin, R., "Pathogenic Microbes and Disease: Causation or Consequences?" April 2020.

Olshansky, S. Jay, Douglas Passaro, Ronald C. Hershow, Jennifer Layden, Bruce A. Carnes, Jacob Brody, Leonard Hayflick, Robert N. Butler, David B. Allison, and David S. Ludwig. "A Potential Decline in Life Expectancy in the United States in the 21st Century." *The New England Journal of Medicine* 352 (2005). https://1ref.us/1r7.

Ornish, Dean. *Love and Survival: The Scientific Basis for the Healing Power of Intimacy.* New York, NY: HarperCollins, 1998.

Ott, John. *Health and Light.* New York, NY: Pocket Books, 2000.

Patlak, M. U.S. Department of Health and Human Services. National Institutes of Health and National Heart, Lung and Blood Institute. "Your Guide to Healthy Sleep." NIH Publication No. 11-5271, November 2005. Revised August 2011.

Perl, James. *Sleep Right in Five Nights: a clear and effective guide for conquering insomnia.* New York, NY: William Morrow and Company, Inc., 1993.

Raman, Ryan. "How to Safely Get Vitamin D From Sunlight." healthline. https://1ref.us/1qm.

Richling, Carra. "Plant-Based Eating: Getting the Right Nutrition." ornish lifestyle medicine. https://1ref.us/1qx.

Rohn, Jim. *The Treasury of Quotes.* Southlake, TX: Jim Rohn International, 2006.

Salford, L. G. Salford, et al. "Permeability of the blood-brain barrier induced by 915 MHz electromagnetic radiation, continuous wave and modulated at 8, 16, 50, and 200 Hz." *Microscopic Research Technology* 27, (1994).

Saltzman, John R., reviewing Peery AF et al. Burden and cost of gastrointestinal, liver and pancreatic diseases in the United States. *Gastroenterology*. https://1ref.us/1qz.

Seligman, Martin. *Learned Optimism.* New York, NY: Picket Books, 1998.

Shapiro, Fred R. *The Yale Book of Quotations.* New Haven, CT: Yale University Press, 2006.

Siegel, B. *Love, Medicine & Miracles: Lessons Learned About Self-Healing from a Surgeon's Experience with Exceptional Patients.* New York, NY: Harper Perennial, 1986.

Sitwell, Kamila Laura. "Sugar consumption now vs 100 years ago." https://1ref.us/1r8.

Smirnov, Igor. "Electromagnetic Radiation Optimum Neutralizer." *Explore Magazine,* 2002.

Smirnov, I. V. "The Exposure of Normal Human Astrocytes Cells to Mobile Phone Radiation with and without MRET-Nylon Protection." *European Journal of Scientific Research* 37, no. 2 (2009).

Sokal, Karol, and Pawel Sokal. "Earthing the human body influences physiologic processes." NCBI. https://1ref.us/1qo.

Spiegel, K. et al. "Sleep curtailment in healthy young men is associated with decreased levels of leptin, elevated ghrelin levels, and increased hunger and appetite." *Annals of Internal Medicine* 141, no. 11 (2004).

Srikanthan, Preethi, and Arun Karlamangla. "Muscle Mass Index as a Predictor of Longevity in Older-Adults." *The American Journal of Medicine* 127, no. 6 (2014).

Swindoll, Charles R. goodreads. https://1ref.us/1rm.

Tartakovsky, Margarita. "8 Keys to a Strong Relationship." https://1ref.us/1rv.

"The health benefits of strong relationships." Harvard Health Publishing. Harvard Medical School. https://1ref.us/1ru.

"The pros and cons of organic foods." Jen's Modest Treasures. https://1ref.us/1r5.

The Rolling Stones, Jagger-Richards. "Honky Tonk Women." June 1969; London Records (US), released July 4, 1969, as a non-album single.

Thurman, Howard. *The Living Wisdom of Howard Thurman: A Visionary for Our Time.* Sounds True Publishing, 2010.

U.S. Environmental Protection Agency. 1987. "The total exposure assessment methodology (TEAM) study: Summary and analysis." EPA/600/6-87/002a. Washington, DC.

"Vitamin B12." National Institutes of Health. https://1ref.us/1re.

"Vitamin D and Diabetes." Diabetes.co.uk. https://1ref.us/1rb.

Voth, David M. *The 10 Secrets Revenue Canada Doesn't Want You to Know.* Saskatoon, SK, CA: Voth Publications, 1996.

Wertheimer, Nancy, and Ed Leeper. "Adult cancer related to electrical wires near the home." *International Journal of Epidemiology* 11 (1982).

Wadyka, Sally. "How to Get the Biggest Benefits of Walking." *Consumer Reports*. https://1ref.us/1ql.

West, Helen. "9 Signs and Symptoms of Vitamin B12 Deficiency." healthline. https://1ref.us/1rf.

White, Ellen G. *Christ's Object Lessons.* Washington, DC: Review and Herald Publishing Association, 1900.

———. *Education.* Mountain View, CA: Pacific Press, 1903.

———. *The Adventist Home.* Hagerstown, MD: Review and Herald Publishing Association, 1952.

———. *The Desire of Ages.* Mountain View, CA: Pacific Press Publishing Association, 1898.

———. *The Ministry of Healing.* Mountain View, CA: Pacific Press Publishing Association, 1905.

Wilks, James. *The Game Changers*. Directed by Louie Psihoyos: September 16, 2019 (Germany). https://1ref.us/1qv.

Wingard, Deborah, and Lisa Berkman, et al. "Mortality risk associated with sleeping patterns among adults." *Sleep* 6, no. 2 (1983).

"Why is love so important?" *The Economic Times*. https://1ref.us/1rs.

"Why Is Vitamin D So Important for Your Health?" HCP Live. https://1ref.us/1rc.

Yang, Sarah. "Human security at risk as depletion of soil accelerates, scientists warn." Berkeley News. https://1ref.us/1ra.

Youngstedt, Shawn. "Has Adult Sleep Duration Declined Over the Last 50+ Years?" NCBI. https://1ref.us/1qf.

"Zig Ziglar Quotable Quote." goodreads. https://1ref.us/1ro.

TEACH Services, Inc.
P U B L I S H I N G

We invite you to view the complete
selection of titles we publish at:
www.TEACHServices.com

We encourage you to write us
with your thoughts about this,
or any other book we publish at:
info@TEACHServices.com

TEACH Services' titles may be purchased in
bulk quantities for educational, fund-raising,
business, or promotional use.
bulksales@TEACHServices.com

Finally, if you are interested in seeing
your own book in print, please contact us at:
publishing@TEACHServices.com
We are happy to review your manuscript at no charge.

CPSIA information can be obtained
at www.ICGtesting.com
Printed in the USA
BVHW060447160322
631580BV00002B/9